Virtual Clinical Excursions—Obstetrics-Pediatrics

for

Perry, Hockenberry, Lowdermilk, and Wilson:
Maternal Child Nursing Care,
5th Edition

Virtual Clinical Excursions—Obstetrics-Pediatrics

for

Perry, Hockenberry, Lowdermilk, and Wilson: Maternal Child Nursing Care, 5th Edition

prepared by

Kelly Ann Crum, RN, MSN
Chair, Department of Nursing
Associate Professor
Maranatha Baptist Bible College
Watertown, Wisconsin

Certified Advanced Facilitator
University of Phoenix
Phoenix, Arizona

David Wilson, MS, RNC
Staff, Children's Day Hospital
St. Francis Hospital
Tulsa, Oklahoma

software developed by

Wolfsong Informatics, LLC
Tucson, Arizona

ELSEVIER
MOSBY

ELSEVIER
MOSBY

3251 Riverport Lane
Maryland Heights, Missouri 63043

VIRTUAL CLINICAL EXCURSIONS—OBSTETRIC-PEDIATRIC FOR
PERRY, HOCKENBERRY, LOWDERMILK, AND WILSON:
MATERNAL CHILD NURSING CARE
FIFTH EDITION

ISBN: 978-0-323-22187-0

Copyright © 2014, 2010, 2006 by Mosby, Inc., an imprint of Elsevier Inc.

Notice

Knowledge and best practice in this field are constantly changing. As new research and experience
broaden our understanding, changes in research methods, professional practices, or medical treatment may become necessary.
Practitioners and researchers must always rely on their own experience and knowledge in evaluating and using any information, methods, compounds, or experiments described herein. In using
such information or methods they should be mindful of their own safety and the safety of others,
including parties for whom they have a professional responsibility.
With respect to any drug or pharmaceutical products identified, readers are advised to check the
most current information provided (i) on procedures featured or (ii) by the manufacturer of each
product to be administered, to verify the recommended dose or formula, the method and duration
of administration, and contraindications. It is the responsibility of practitioners, relying on their
own experience and knowledge of their patients, to make diagnoses, to determine dosages and the
best treatment for each individual patient, and to take all appropriate safety precautions.
To the fullest extent of the law, neither the Publisher nor the authors, contributors, or editors,
assume any liability for any injury and/or damage to persons or property as a matter of products
liability, negligence or otherwise, or from any use or operation of any methods, products, instructions, or ideas contained in the material herein.

ISBN: 978-0-323-22187-0

Director, Simulation Solutions: *Jeff Downing*
Content Development Specialist: *Angela Perdue*
Content Coordinator: *Khori Wright*
Senior Project Manager: *Tracey Schriefer*
Publishing Services Manager: *Jeff Patterson*

Printed in the United States of America

Last digit is the print number: 9   8   7   6   5   4   3   2   1

Kim D. Cooper, MSN, RN
Dean, School of Nursing
Ivy Tech Community College
Terre Haute, Indiana

Kelly Ann Crum, MSN, RN
Chair, Department of Nursing
Associate Professor
Maranatha Baptist Bible College
Watertown, Wisconsin

Certified Advanced Facilitator
University of Phoenix
Phoenix, Arizona

Susan Fertig McDonald, DNP, RN, CS
Clinical Nurse Specialist—Psychiatry
VA San Diego Healthcare System
San Diego, California

Kristin Ulstad Propson, MN, RN
Decorah, Iowa

Jeffrey L. Wagner, PharmD, MPH, RPh, BCPS
Assistant Director
Department of Pharmacy
Texas Children's Hospital
Houston, Texas

Textbook

Shannon E. Perry, RN, CNS, PhD, FAAN
Professor Emerita, School of Nursing
San Francisco State University
San Francisco, California

Marilyn J. Hockenberry, PhD, RN-CS, PNP, FAAN
Bessie Baker Distinguished Professor of Nursing and Professor of Pediatrics
Chair, Duke Institutional Review Board
Duke University
Durham, North Carolina

Deitra Leonard Lowdermilk, RNC, PhD, FAAN
Clinical Professor, Emerita
University of North Carolina at Chapel Hill
Chapel Hill, North Carolina

David Wilson, MS, RNC
Staff, Children's Day Hospital
St. Francis Hospital
Tulsa, Oklahoma

Kitty Cashion, RN-BC, MSN
Clinical Nurse Specialist
Department of Obstetrics and Gynecology
Division of Maternal-Fetal Medicine
University of Tennessee Health Science Center
Memphis, Tennessee

Kathryn Alden, RN, MSN, EdD, IBCLC
Clinical Associate Professor
School of Nursing
University of North Carolina at Chapel Hill
Chapel Hill, North Carolina

Table of Contents
Virtual Clinical Excursions Workbook

Table of Contents
Perry, Hockenberry, Lowdermilk, and Wilson:
Maternal Child Nursing Care, 5th Edition

Getting Started

GETTING SET UP WITH VCE ONLINE ───────────────────

The product you have purchased is part of the Evolve Learning System. Please read the following information thoroughly to get started.

■ HOW TO ACCESS YOUR VCE RESOURCES ON EVOLVE

There are two ways to access your VCE Resources on Evolve:

1. If your instructor has enrolled you in your VCE Evolve Resources, you will receive an email with your registration details.

2. If your instructor has asked you to self-enroll in your VCE Evolve Resources, he or she will provide you with your Course ID (for example, 1479_jdoe73_0001). You will then need to follow the instructions at https://evolve.elsevier.com/cs/studentEnroll.html.

■ HOW TO ACCESS THE ONLINE VIRTUAL HOSPITAL

The online virtual hospital is available through the Evolve VCE Resources. There is no software to download or install: the online virtual hospital runs within your internet browser, using a pop-up window.

■ TECHNICAL REQUIREMENTS

- Broadband connection (DSL or cable)
- 1024 x 768 screen resolution
- Mozilla Firefox 18.0, Internet Explorer 9.0, Google Chrome, or Safari 5 (or higher)
  Note: Pop-up blocking software/settings must be disabled.
- Adobe Acrobat Reader
- Additional technical requirements available at http://evolvesupport.elsevier.com

■ HOW TO ACCESS THE WORKBOOK

There are two ways to access the workbook portion of *Virtual Clinical Excursions:*

1. Print workbook
2. An electronic version of the workbook, available within the VCE Evolve Resources

■ TECHNICAL SUPPORT

Technical support for *Virtual Clinical Excursions* is available by visiting the Technical Support Center at http://evolvesupport.elsevier.com or by calling 1-800-222-9570 inside the United States and Canada.

Trademarks: Windows® and Macintosh® are registered trademarks.

A QUICK TOUR

Welcome to *Virtual Clinical Excursions—Obstetrics-Pediatrics*, a virtual hospital setting in which you can work with multiple complex patient simulations and also learn to access and evaluate the information resources that are essential for high-quality patient care. The virtual hospital, Pacific View Regional Hospital, has realistic architecture and access to patient rooms, a Nurses' Station, and a Medication Room.

■ BEFORE YOU START

Make sure you have your textbook nearby when you use *Virtual Clinical Excursions*. You will want to consult topic areas in your textbook frequently while working with the virtual hospital and workbook.

■ HOW TO SIGN IN

- Enter your name on the Student Nurse identification badge.
- Next, click the down arrow next to **Select Floor**. For this quick tour, choose **Obstetrics**.
- Now click the down arrow next to **Select Period of Care**. This drop-down menu gives you four periods of care from which to choose. In Periods of Care 1 through 3, you can actively engage in patient assessment, entry of data in the electronic patient record (EPR), and medication administration. Period of Care 4 presents the day in review. Highlight and click the appropriate period of care. (For this quick tour, choose **Period of Care 1: 0730-0815**.)
- Click **Go**. This takes you to the Patient List screen (see the *How to Select a Patient* section below). Note that the virtual time is provided in the box at the lower left corner of the screen (0730, since we chose Period of Care 1).

Note: If you choose to work during Period of Care 4: 1900-2000, the Patient List screen is skipped since you are not able to visit patients or administer medications during the shift. Instead, you are taken directly to the Nurses' Station, where the records of all the patients on the floor are available for your review.

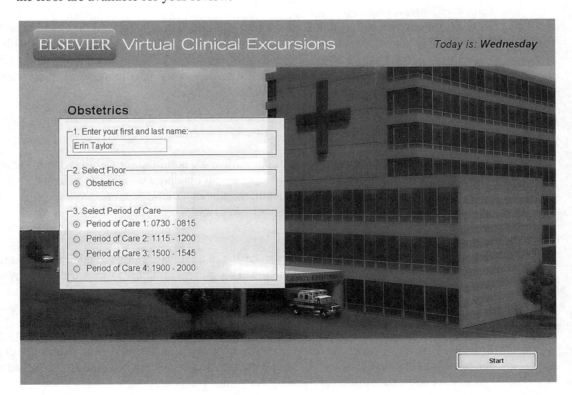

■ PATIENT LIST

OBSTETRICS UNIT

Dorothy Grant (Room 201)
30-week intrauterine pregnancy—A 25-year-old multipara Caucasian female admitted with abdominal trauma following a domestic violence incident. Her complications include preterm labor and extensive social issues such as acquiring safe housing for her family upon discharge.

Stacey Crider (Room 202)
27-week intrauterine pregnancy—A 21-year-old primigravida Native American female admitted for intravenous tocolysis, bacterial vaginosis, and poorly controlled insulin-dependent gestational diabetes. Strained family relationships and social isolation complicate this patient's ability to comply with strict dietary requirements and prenatal care.

Kelly Brady (Room 203)
26-week intrauterine pregnancy—A 35-year-old primigravida Caucasian female urgently admitted for progressive symptoms of preeclampsia. A history of inadequate coping with major life stressors leave her at risk for a recurrence of depression as she faces a diagnosis of HELLP syndrome and the delivery of a severely premature infant.

Maggie Gardner (Room 204)
22-week intrauterine pregnancy—A 41-year-old multigravida African-American female admitted for a high-risk pregnancy evaluation and rule out diagnosis of systemic lupus erythematosus. Coping with chronic pain, fatigue, and a history of multiple miscarriages contribute to an anxiety disorder and the need for social service intervention.

Gabriela Valenzuela (Room 205)
34-week intrauterine pregnancy—A 21-year-old primigravida Hispanic female with a history of mitral valve prolapse admitted for uterine cramping and vaginal bleeding suggestive of placental abruption following an unrestrained motor vehicle accident. Her needs include staff support for an unprepared-for labor and possible preterm birth.

Laura Wilson (Room 206)
37-week intrauterine pregnancy—An 18-year-old primigravida Caucasian female urgently admitted after being found unconscious at home. Her complications include HIV-positive status and chronic polysubstance abuse. Unrealistic expectations of parenthood and living with a chronic illness combined with strained family relations prompt comprehensive social and psychiatric evaluations initiated on the day of simulation.

PEDIATRICS UNIT

George Gonzalez (Room 301)
Diabetic ketoacidosis—An 11-year-old Hispanic male admitted for stabilization of blood glucose level and diabetic re-education associated with his diagnosis of type 1 diabetes mellitus. This patient's poor compliance with insulin therapy and dietary regime have resulted in frequent and repeated hospital admissions for diabetic ketoacidosis.

Tommy Douglas (Room 302)
Traumatic brain injury—A 6-year-old Caucasian male transferred from the Pediatric Intensive Care Unit in preparation for organ donation. This patient is status post ventriculostomy with negative intracerebral blood flow and requires extensive hemodynamic monitoring and support, along with compassionate family care.

Carrie Richards (Room 303)
Bronchiolitis—A 3½-month-old African-American female admitted with respiratory distress due to respiratory syncytial virus, along with dehydration and an inadequate nutritional status. Parent education and support are among her primary needs.

Stephanie Brown (Room 304)

Meningitis—A 3-year-old African-American female with a history of spastic cerebral palsy admitted for intravenous antibiotic therapy, neurologic monitoring, and support for a diagnosis of acute meningitis. Maintenance of physical and occupational programs addressing her mobility limitations complicate her acute care stay.

Tiffany Sheldon (Room 305)

Anorexia nervosa—A 14-year-old Caucasian female admitted for dehydration, electrolyte imbalance, and malnutrition following a syncope episode at home. This patient has a history of eating disorders, which have resulted in multiple hospital admissions and strained family dynamics between mother and daughter.

■ HOW TO SELECT A PATIENT

- You can choose one or more patients to work with from the Patient List by checking the box to the left of the patient name(s). For this quick tour, select Dorothy Grant. (In order to receive a scorecard for a patient, the patient must be selected before proceeding to the Nurses' Station.)
- Click on **Get Report** to the right of the medical records number (MRN) to view a summary of the patient's care during the 12-hour period before your arrival on the unit.
- After reviewing the report, click on **Go to Nurses' Station** in the right lower corner to begin your care. (*Note:* If you have been assigned to care for multiple patients, you can click on **Return to Patient List** to select and review the report for each additional patient before going to the Nurses' Station.)

Note: Even though the Patient List is initially skipped when you sign in to work for Period of Care 4, you can still access this screen if you wish to review the shift report for any of the patients. To do so, simply click on **Patient List** near the top left corner of the Nurses' Station (or click on the clipboard to the left of the Kardex). Then click on **Get Report** for the patient(s) whose care you are reviewing. This may be done during any period of care.

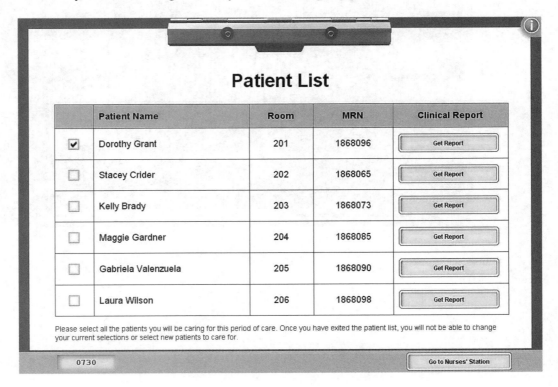

Patient List

	Patient Name	Room	MRN	Clinical Report
☑	Dorothy Grant	201	1868096	Get Report
☐	Stacey Crider	202	1868065	Get Report
☐	Kelly Brady	203	1868073	Get Report
☐	Maggie Gardner	204	1868085	Get Report
☐	Gabriela Valenzuela	205	1868090	Get Report
☐	Laura Wilson	206	1868098	Get Report

Please select all the patients you will be caring for this period of care. Once you have exited the patient list, you will not be able to change your current selections or select new patients to care for.

0730   Go to Nurses' Station

■ HOW TO FIND A PATIENT'S RECORDS

NURSES' STATION

Within the Nurses' Station, you will see:

1. A clipboard that contains the patient list for that floor.
2. A chart rack with patient charts labeled by room number, a notebook labeled Kardex, and a notebook labeled MAR (Medication Administration Record).
3. A desktop computer with access to the Electronic Patient Record (EPR).
4. A tool bar across the top of the screen that can also be used to access the Patient List, EPR, Chart, MAR, and Kardex. This tool bar is also accessible from each patient's room.
5. A Drug Guide containing information about the medications you are able to administer to your patients.
6. A Laboratory Guide containing normal value ranges for all laboratory tests you may come across in the virtual patient hospital.
7. A tool bar across the bottom of the screen that can be used to access the Floor Map, patient rooms, Medication Room, and Drug Guide.

As you run your cursor over an item, it will be highlighted. To select, simply click on the item. As you use these resources, you will always be able to return to the Nurses' Station by clicking on the **Return to Nurses' Station** bar located in the right lower corner of your screen.

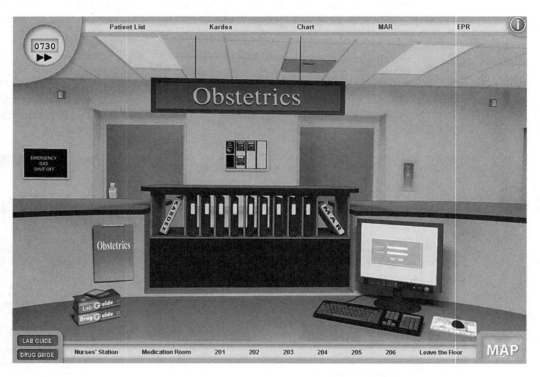

MEDICATION ADMINISTRATION RECORD (MAR)

The MAR icon located on the tool bar at the top of your screen accesses current 24-hour medications for each patient. Click on the icon and the MAR will open. (*Note:* You can also access the MAR by clicking on the MAR notebook on the far right side of the book rack in the center of the screen.) Within the MAR, tabs on the right side of the screen allow you to select patients by room number. Be careful to make sure you select the correct tab number for *your* patient rather than simply reading the first record that appears after the MAR opens. Each MAR sheet lists the following:

- Medications
- Route and dosage of each medication
- Times of administration of each medication

Note: The MAR changes each day. Expired MARs are stored in the patients' charts.

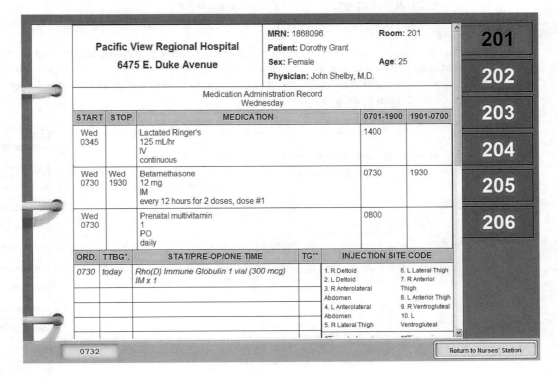

Charts

To access patient charts, either click on the **Chart** icon at the top of your screen or anywhere within the chart rack in the center of the Nurses' Station screen. When the close-up view appears, the individual charts are labeled by room number. To open a chart, click on the room number of the patient whose chart you wish to review. The patient's name and allergies will appear on the left side of the screen, along with a list of tabs on the right side of the screen, allowing you to view the following data:

- Allergies
- Physician's Orders
- Physician's Notes
- Nurse's Notes
- Laboratory Reports
- Diagnostic Reports
- Surgical Reports
- Consultations
- Patient Education
- History and Physical
- Nursing Admission
- Expired MARs
- Consents
- Mental Health
- Admissions
- Emergency Department

Information appears in real time. The entries are in reverse chronologic order, so use the down arrow at the right side of each chart page to scroll down to view previous entries. Flip from tab to tab to view multiple data fields or click on **Return to Nurses' Station** in the lower right corner of the screen to exit the chart.

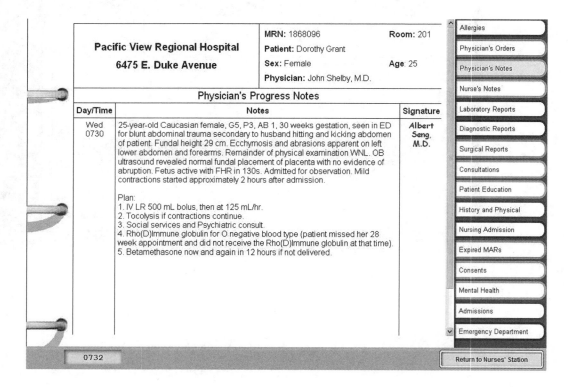

ELECTRONIC PATIENT RECORD (EPR)

The EPR can be accessed from the computer in the Nurses' Station or from the EPR icon located in the tool bar at the top of your screen. To access a patient's EPR:

- Click on either the computer screen or the **EPR** icon.
- Your username and password are automatically filled in.
- Click on **Login** to enter the EPR.
- *Note:* Like the MAR, the EPR is arranged numerically. Thus when you enter, you are initially shown the records of the patient in the lowest room number on the floor. To view the correct data for *your* patient, remember to select the correct room number, using the dropdown menu for the Patient field at the top left corner of the screen.

The EPR used in Pacific View Regional Hospital represents a composite of commercial versions being used in hospitals. You can access the EPR:

- to review existing data for a patient (by room number).
- to enter data you collect while working with a patient.

The EPR is updated daily, so no matter what day or part of a shift you are working, there will be a current EPR with the patient's data from the past days of the current hospital stay. This type of simulated EPR allows you to examine how data for different attributes have changed over time, as well as to examine data for all of a patient's attributes at a particular time. The EPR is fully functional (as it is in a real-life hospital). You can enter such data as blood pressure, breath sounds, and certain treatments. The EPR will not, however, allow you to enter data for a previous time period. Use the arrows at the bottom of the screen to move forward and backward in time.

Patient: 201	Category: Vital Signs			**0735**	
Name: Dorothy Grant	**Wed 0700**	**Wed 0715**	**Wed 0733**	**Code Meanings**	
PAIN: LOCATION	A			A	Abdomen
PAIN: RATING	1-2			Ar	Arm
PAIN: CHARACTERISTICS	I			B	Back
PAIN: VOCAL CUES				C	Chest
PAIN: FACIAL CUES				Ft	Foot
PAIN: BODILY CUES				H	Head
PAIN: SYSTEM CUES				Hd	Hand
PAIN: FUNCTIONAL EFFECTS				L	Left
PAIN: PREDISPOSING FACTORS				Lg	Leg
PAIN: RELIEVING FACTORS				Lw	Lower
PCA				N	Neck
TEMPERATURE (F)	98.2			NN	See Nurses notes
TEMPERATURE (C)				OS	Operative site
MODE OF MEASUREMENT	O			Or	See Physicians orders
SYSTOLIC PRESSURE	126			PN	See Progress notes
DIASTOLIC PRESSURE	68			R	Right
BP MODE OF MEASUREMENT	NIBP			Up	Upper
HEART RATE	70				
RESPIRATORY RATE	18				
SpO2 (%)	96				
BLOOD GLUCOSE					
WEIGHT					
HEIGHT					

Return to Nurses' Station

At the top of the EPR screen, you can choose patients by their room numbers. In addition, you have access to 17 different categories of patient data. To change patients or data categories, click the down arrow to the right of the room number or category.

The categories of patient data in the EPR are as follows:

- Vital Signs
- Respiratory
- Cardiovascular
- Neurologic
- Gastrointestinal
- Excretory
- Musculoskeletal
- Integumentary
- Reproductive
- Psychosocial
- Wounds and Drains
- Activity
- Hygiene and Comfort
- Safety
- Nutrition
- IV
- Intake and Output

Remember, each hospital selects its own codes. The codes used in the EPR at Pacific View Regional Hospital may be different from ones you have seen in your clinical rotations. Take some time to acquaint yourself with the codes. Within the Vital Signs category, click on any item in the left column (e.g., Pain: Characteristics). In the far-right column, you will see a list of code meanings for the possible findings and/or descriptors for that assessment area.

You will use the codes to record the data you collect as you work with patients. Click on the box in the last time column to the right of any item and wait for the code meanings applicable to that entry to appear. Select the appropriate code to describe your assessment findings and type it in the box. (*Note:* If no cursor appears within the box, click on the box again until the blue shading disappears and the blinking cursor appears.) Once the data are typed in this box, they are entered into the patient's record for this period of care only.

To leave the EPR, click on **Exit EPR** in the bottom right corner of the screen.

■ **VISITING A PATIENT**

From the Nurses' Station, click on the room number of the patient you wish to visit (in the tool bar at the bottom of your screen). Once you are inside the room, you will see a still photo of your patient in the top left corner. To verify that this is the correct patient, click on the **Check Armband** icon to the right of the photo. The patient's identification data will appear. If you click on **Check Allergies** (the next icon to the right), a list of the patient's allergies (if any) will replace the photo.

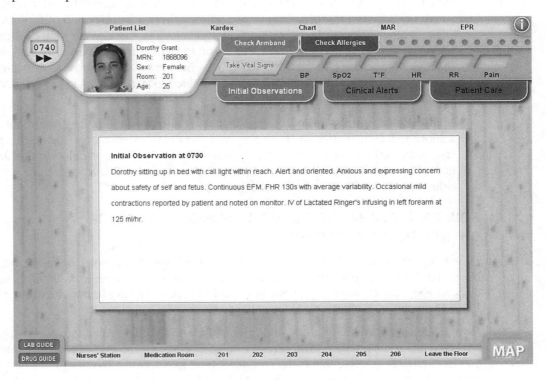

Also located in the patient's room are multiple icons you can use to assess the patient or the patient's medications. A virtual clock is provided in the upper left corner of the room to monitor your progress in real time. (*Note:* The fast-forward icon within the virtual clock will advance the time by 2-minute intervals when clicked.)

- The tool bar across the top of the screen allows you to check the **Patient List**, access the **EPR** to check or enter data, and view the patient's **Chart**, **MAR**, or **Kardex**.

- The **Take Vital Signs** icon allows you to measure the patient's up-to-the-minute blood pressure, oxygen saturation, temperature, heart rate, respiratory rate, and pain level.

- Each time you enter a patient's room, you are given an Initial Observation report to review (in the text box under the patient's photo). These notes are provided to give you a "look" at the patient as if you had just stepped into the room. You can also click on the **Initial Observations** icon to return to this box from other views within the patient's room. To the right of this icon is **Clinical Alerts**, a resource that allows you to make decisions about priority medication interventions based on emerging data collected in real time. Check this screen throughout your period of care to avoid missing critical information related to recently ordered or STAT medications.

- Clicking on **Patient Care** opens up three specific learning environments within the patient room: **Physical Assessment**, **Nurse-Client Interactions**, and **Medication Administration**.

- To perform a **Physical Assessment**, choose a body area (such as **Head & Neck**) from the column of yellow buttons. This activates a list of system subcategories for that body area (e.g., see **Sensory**, **Neurologic**, etc. in the green boxes). After you select the system you wish to evaluate, a brief description of the assessment findings will appear in a box to the right. A still photo provides a "snapshot" of how an assessment of this area might be done or what the finding might look like. For every body area, you can also click on **Equipment** on the right side of the screen.

- To the right of the Physical Assessment icon is **Nurse-Client Interactions**. Clicking on this icon will reveal the times and titles of any videos available for viewing. (*Note:* If the video you wish to see is not listed, this means you have not yet reached the correct virtual time to view that video. Check the virtual clock; you may return to access the video once its designated time has occurred—as long as you do so within the same period of care. Or you can click on the fast-forward icon within the virtual clock to advance the time by 2-minute intervals. You will then need to click again on **Patient Care** and **Nurse-Client Interactions** to refresh the screen.) To view a listed video, click on the white arrow to the right of the video title. Use the control buttons below the video to start, stop, pause, rewind, or fast-forward the action or to mute the sound.

- **Medication Administration** is the pathway that allows you to review and administer medications to a patient after you have prepared them in the Medication Room. This process is also addressed further in the *How to Prepare Medications* section below and in *Medications* in the **Detailed Tour**. For additional hands-on practice, see *Reducing Medication Errors* below the **Quick Tour** and **Detailed Tour** in your resources.

■ HOW TO QUIT, CHANGE PATIENTS, CHANGE FLOORS, OR CHANGE PERIODS OF CARE

How to Quit: From most screens, you may click the **Leave the Floor** icon on the bottom tool bar to the right of the patient room numbers. (*Note:* From some screens, you will first need to click an **Exit** button or **Return to Nurses' Station** before clicking **Leave the Floor**.) When the Floor Menu appears, click **Exit** to leave the program.

How to Change Patients, Floors, or Periods of Care: To change patients, simply click on the new patient's room number. (You cannot receive a scorecard for a new patient, however, unless you have already selected that patient on the Patient List screen.) To change to a new period of care, to change floors, or to restart the virtual clock, click on **Leave the Floor** and then on **Restart the Program**.

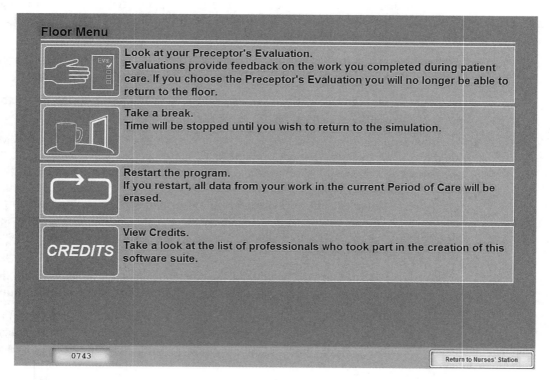

■ HOW TO PREPARE MEDICATIONS

From the Nurses' Station or the patient's room, you can access the Medication Room by clicking on the icon in the tool bar at the bottom of your screen to the left of the patient room numbers.

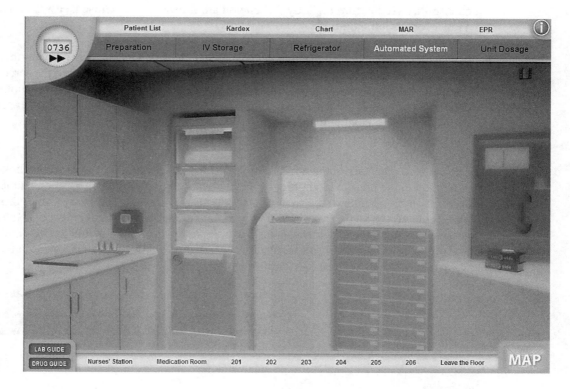

In the Medication Room you have access to the following (from left to right):

- A preparation area is located on the counter under the cabinets. To begin the medication preparation process, click on the tray on the counter or click on the **Preparation** icon at the top of the screen. The next screen leads you through a specific sequence (called the Preparation Wizard) to prepare medications one at a time for administration to a patient. However, no medication has been selected at this time. We will do this while working with a patient in *A Detailed Tour*. To exit this screen, click on **View Medication Room**.

- To the right of the cabinets (and above the refrigerator), IV storage bins are provided. Click on the bins themselves or on the **IV Storage** icon at the top of the screen. The bins are labeled **Microinfusion**, **Small Volume**, and **Large Volume**. Click on an individual bin to see a list of its contents. If you needed to prepare an IV medication at this time, you could click on the medication and its label would appear to the right under the patient's name. (*Note:* You can **Open** and **Close** any medication label by clicking the appropriate icon.) Next, you would click **Put Medication on Tray**. If you ever change your mind or decide that you have put the incorrect medication on the tray, you can reverse your actions by highlighting the medication on the tray and then clicking **Put Medication in Bin**. Click **Close Bin** in the right bottom corner to exit. **View Medication Room** brings you back to a full view of the entire room.

- A refrigerator is located under the IV storage bins to hold any medications that must be stored below room temperature. Click on the refrigerator door or on the **Refrigerator** icon at the top of the screen. Then click on the close-up view of the door to access the medications. When you are finished, click **Close Door** and then **View Medication Room**.

- To prepare controlled substances, click the **Automated System** icon at the top of the screen or click the computer monitor located to the right of the IV storage bins. A login screen will appear; your name and password are automatically filled in. Click **Login**. Select the patient for whom you wish to access medications; then select the correct medication drawer to open (they are stored alphabetically). Click **Open Drawer**, highlight the proper medication, and choose **Put Medication on Tray**. When you are finished, click **Close Drawer** and then **View Medication Room**.

- Next to the Automated System is a set of drawers identified by patient room number. To access these, click on the drawers or on the **Unit Dosage** icon at the top of the screen. This provides a close-up view of the drawers. To open a drawer, click on the room number of the patient you are working with. Next, click on the medication you would like to prepare for the patient, and a label will appear, listing the medication strength, units, and dosage per unit. To exit, click **Close Drawer**; then click **View Medication Room**.

At any time, you can learn about a medication you wish to prepare for a patient by clicking on the **Drug** icon in the bottom left corner of the medication room screen or by clicking the **Drug Guide** book on the counter to the right of the unit dosage drawers. The **Drug Guide** provides information about the medications commonly included in nursing drug handbooks. Nutritional supplements and maintenance intravenous fluid preparations are not included. Highlight a medication in the alphabetical list; relevant information about the drug will appear in the screen below. To exit, click **Return to Medication Room**.

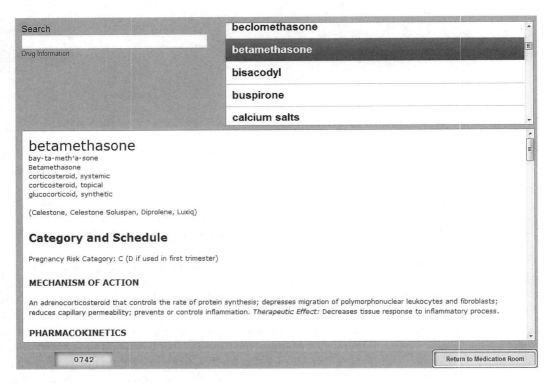

To access the MAR from the Medication Room and to review the medications ordered for a patient, click on the **MAR** icon located in the tool bar at the top of your screen and then click on the correct tab for your patient's room number. You may also click the **Review MAR** icon in the tool bar at the bottom of your screen from inside each medication storage area.

After you have chosen and prepared medications, go to the patient's room to administer them by clicking on the room number in the bottom tool bar. Inside the patient's room, click **Patient Care** and then **Medication Administration** and follow the proper administration sequence.

■ PRECEPTOR'S EVALUATIONS

When you have finished a session, click on **Leave the Floor** to go to the Floor Menu. At this point, you can click on the top icon (**Look at Your Preceptor's Evaluation**) to receive a score-card that provides feedback on the work you completed during patient care.

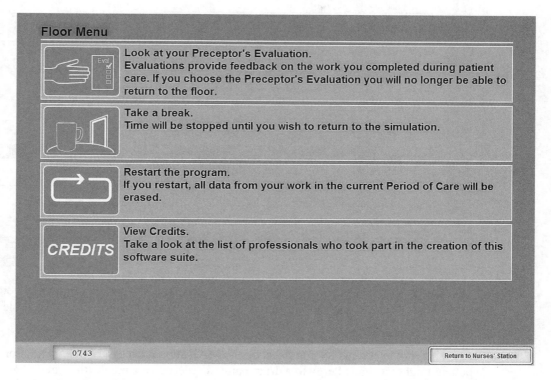

Evaluations are available for each patient you selected when you signed in for the current period of care. Click on the **Medication Scorecard** icon to see an example.

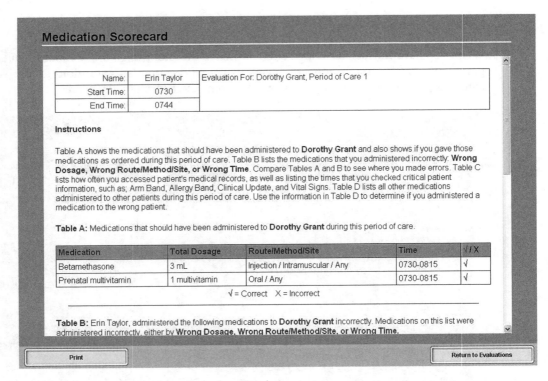

Medication Scorecard

Name:	Erin Taylor	Evaluation For: Dorothy Grant, Period of Care 1
Start Time:	0730	
End Time:	0744	

Instructions

Table A shows the medications that should have been administered to **Dorothy Grant** and also shows if you gave those medications as ordered during this period of care. Table B lists the medications that you administered incorrectly: **Wrong Dosage, Wrong Route/Method/Site, or Wrong Time**. Compare Tables A and B to see where you made errors. Table C lists how often you accessed patient's medical records, as well as listing the times that you checked critical patient information, such as; Arm Band, Allergy Band, Clinical Update, and Vital Signs. Table D lists all other medications administered to other patients during this period of care. Use the information in Table D to determine if you administered a medication to the wrong patient.

Table A: Medications that should have been administered to **Dorothy Grant** during this period of care.

Medication	Total Dosage	Route/Method/Site	Time	√ / X
Betamethasone	3 mL	Injection / Intramuscular / Any	0730-0815	√
Prenatal multivitamin	1 multivitamin	Oral / Any	0730-0815	√

√ = Correct   X = Incorrect

Table B: Erin Taylor, administered the following medications to **Dorothy Grant** incorrectly. Medications on this list were administered incorrectly, either by **Wrong Dosage, Wrong Route/Method/Site, or Wrong Time.**

| Print | | Return to Evaluations |

The scorecard compares the medications you administered to a patient during a period of care with what should have been administered. Table A lists the correct medications. Table B lists any medications that were administered incorrectly.

Remember, not every medication listed on the MAR should necessarily be given. For example, a patient might have an allergy to a drug that was ordered, or a medication might have been improperly transcribed to the MAR. Predetermined medication "errors" embedded within the program challenge you to exercise critical thinking skills and professional judgment when deciding to administer a medication, just as you would in a real hospital. Use all your available resources, such as the patient's chart and the MAR, to make your decision.

Table C lists the resources that were available to assist you in medication administration. It also documents whether and when you accessed these resources. For example, did you check the patient armband or perform a check of vital signs? If so, when?

You can click **Print** to get a copy of this report if needed. When you have finished reviewing the scorecard, click **Return to Evaluations** and then **Return to Menu**.

■ **FLOOR MAP**

To get a general sense of your location within the hospital, you can click on the **Map** icon found in the lower right corner of most of the screens in the *Virtual Clinical Excursions—Obstetrics-Pediatrics* program. (*Note:* If you are following this quick tour step by step, you will need to **Restart the Program** from the Floor Menu, sign in again, and go to the Nurses' Station to access the map.) When you click the **Map** icon, a floor map appears, showing the layout of the floor you are currently on, as well as a directory of the patients and services on that floor. As you move your cursor over the directory list, the location of each room is highlighted on the map (and vice versa). The floor map can be accessed from the Nurses' Station, Medication Room, and each patient's room.

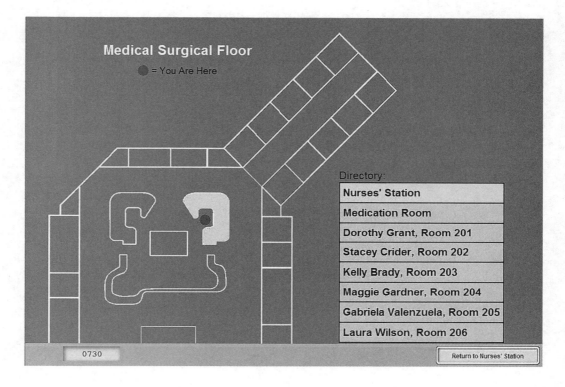

A DETAILED TOUR

If you wish to more thoroughly understand the capabilities of *Virtual Clinical Excursions—Obstetrics-Pediatrics*, take a detailed tour by completing the following section. During this tour, we will work with a specific patient to introduce you to all the different components and learning opportunities available within the software.

■ WORKING WITH A PATIENT

Sign in to work on the Obstetrics Floor for Period of Care 1 (0730-0815). From the Patient List, select Dorothy Grant in Room 201; however, do not go to the Nurses' Station yet.

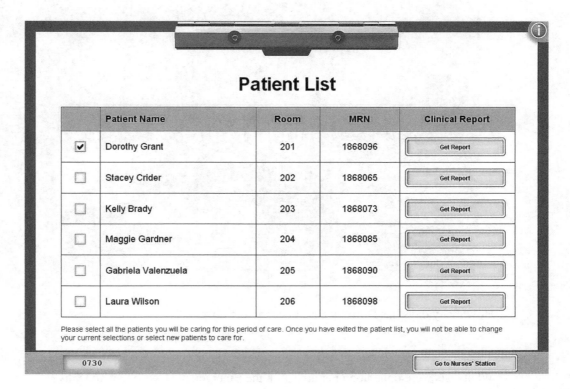

Patient List

	Patient Name	Room	MRN	Clinical Report
☑	Dorothy Grant	201	1868096	Get Report
☐	Stacey Crider	202	1868065	Get Report
☐	Kelly Brady	203	1868073	Get Report
☐	Maggie Gardner	204	1868085	Get Report
☐	Gabriela Valenzuela	205	1868090	Get Report
☐	Laura Wilson	206	1868098	Get Report

Please select all the patients you will be caring for this period of care. Once you have exited the patient list, you will not be able to change your current selections or select new patients to care for.

0730   Go to Nurses' Station

■ REPORT

In hospitals, when one shift ends and another begins, the outgoing nurse who attended a patient will give a verbal and sometimes a written summary of that patient's condition to the incoming nurse who will assume care for the patient. This summary is called a report and is an important source of data to provide an overview of a patient. Your first task is to get the clinical report on Dorothy Grant. To do this, click **Get Report** in the far right column in this patient's row. From a brief review of this summary, identify the problems and areas of concern that you will need to address for this patient.

When you have finished noting any areas of concern, click **Go to Nurses' Station**.

■ CHARTS

You can access Dorothy Grant's chart from the Nurses' Station or from the patient's room (201). From the Nurses' Station, click on the chart rack or on the **Chart** icon in the tool bar at the top of your screen. Next, click on the chart labeled **201** to open the medical record for Dorothy Grant. Click on the **Emergency Department** tab to view a record of why this patient was admitted.

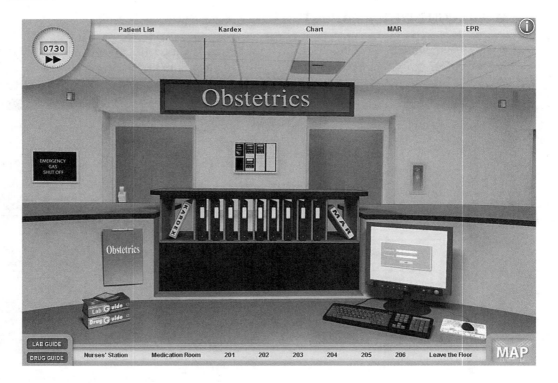

How many days has Dorothy Grant been in the hospital?

What tests were done upon her arrival in the Emergency Department and why?

What was the reason for her admission?

You should also click on **Diagnostic Reports** to learn what additional tests or procedures were performed and when. Finally, review the **Nursing Admission** and **History and Physical** to learn about the health history of this patient. When you are done reviewing the chart, click **Return to Nurses' Station**.

■ MEDICATIONS

Open the Medication Administration Record (MAR) by clicking on the **MAR** icon in the tool bar at the top of your screen. *Remember:* The MAR automatically opens to the first occupied room number on the floor—which is not necessarily your patient's room number! Since you need to access Dorothy Grant's MAR, click on tab **201** (her room number). Always make sure you are giving the *Right Drug to the Right Patient!*

Examine the list of medications ordered for Dorothy Grant. In the table below, list the medications that need to be given during this period of care (0730-0815). For each medication, note the dosage, route, and time to be given.

Time	Medication	Dosage	Route

Click on **Return to Nurses' Station**. Next, click on **201** on the bottom tool bar and then verify that you are indeed in Dorothy Grant's room. Select **Clinical Alerts** (the icon to the right of Initial Observations) to check for any emerging data that might affect your medication administration priorities. Next, go to the patient's chart (click on the **Chart** icon; then click on **201**). When the chart opens, select the **Physician's Orders** tab.

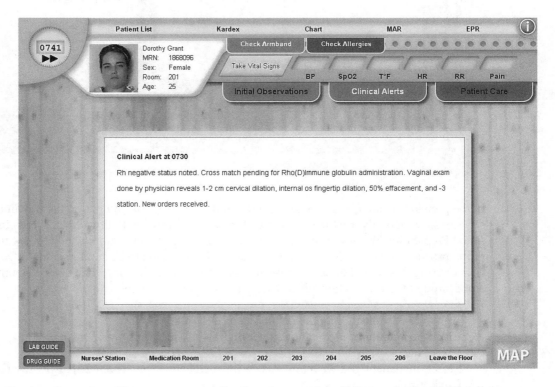

Review the orders. Have any new medications been ordered? Return to the MAR (click **Return to Room 201**; then click **MAR**). Verify that any new medications have been correctly transcribed to the MAR. Mistakes are sometimes made in the transcription process in the hospital setting, and it is sound practice to double-check any new order.

Are there any patient assessments you will need to perform before administering these medications? If so, return to Room 201 and click on **Patient Care** and then **Physical Assessment** to complete those assessments before proceeding.

Now click on the **Medication Room** icon in the tool bar at the bottom of your screen to locate and prepare the medications for Dorothy Grant.

In the Medication Room, you must access the medications for Dorothy Grant from the specific dispensing system in which each medication is stored. Locate each medication that needs to be given in this time period and click on **Put Medication on Tray** as appropriate. (*Hint:* Look in **Unit Dosage** drawer first.) When you are finished, click on **Close Drawer** and then on **View Medication Room**. Now click on the medication tray on the counter on the left side of the medication room screen to begin preparing the medications you have selected. (*Remember:* You can also click **Preparation** in the tool bar at the top of screen.)

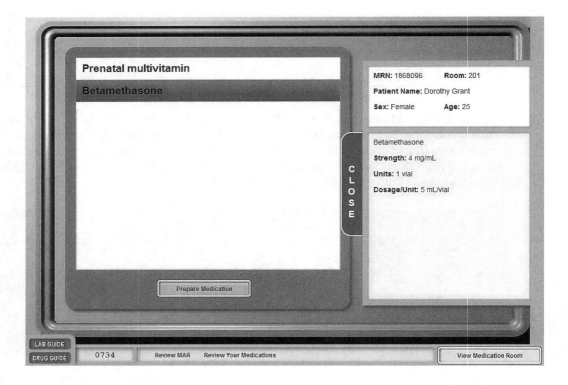

In the preparation area, you should see a list of the medications you put on the tray in the previous steps. Click on the first medication and then click **Prepare**. Follow the onscreen instructions of the Preparation Wizard, providing any data requested. As an example, let's follow the preparation process for betamethasone, one of the medications due to be administered to Dorothy Grant during this period of care. To begin, click on **Betamethasone**; then click **Prepare**. Now work through the Preparation Wizard sequence as detailed below:

> Amount of medication in the ampule: 5 mL.
> Enter the amount of medication you will draw up into a syringe: **3** mL.
> Click **Next**.
> Select the patient you wish to set aside the medication for: **Room 201, Dorothy Grant**.
> Click **Finish**.
> Click **Return to Medication Room**.

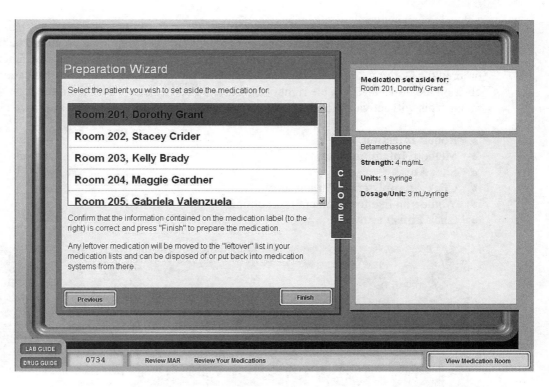

Follow this same basic process for the other medications due to be administered to Dorothy Grant during this period of care. (*Hint:* Look in **IV Storage** and **Automated System**.)

PREPARATION WIZARD EXCEPTIONS

- Some medications in *Virtual Clinical Excursions—Obstetrics-Pediatrics* are prepared by the pharmacy (e.g., IV antibiotics) and taken to the patient room as a whole. This is common practice in most hospitals.
- Blood products are not administered by students through the *Virtual Clinical Excursions—Obstetrics-Pediatrics* simulations since blood administration follows specific protocols not covered in this program.
- The *Virtual Clinical Excursions—Obstetrics-Pediatrics* simulations do not allow for mixing more than one type of medication, such as regular and Lente insulins, in the same syringe. In the clinical setting, when multiple types of insulin are ordered for a patient, the regular insulin is drawn up first, followed by the longer-acting insulin. Insulin is always administered in a special unit-marked syringe.

Now return to Room 201 (click on **201** on the bottom tool bar) to administer Dorothy Grant's medications.

At any time during the medication administration process, you can perform a further review of systems, take vital signs, check information contained within the chart, or verify patient identity and allergies. Inside Dorothy Grant's room, click **Take Vital Signs**. (*Note:* These findings change over time to reflect the temporal changes you would find in a patient similar to Dorothy Grant.)

When you have gathered all the data you need, click on **Patient Care** and then select **Medication Administration**. Any medications you prepared in the previous steps should be listed on the left side of your screen. Let's continue the administration process with the betamethasone ordered for Dorothy Grant. Click to highlight **Betamethasone** in the list of medications. Next, click on the down arrow to the right of **Select** and choose **Administer** from the drop-down menu. This will activate the Administration Wizard. Complete the Wizard sequence as follows:

- Route: **Injection**
- Method: **Intramuscular**
- Site: **Any**
- Click **Administer to Patient** arrow.
- Would you like to document this administration in the MAR? **Yes**
- Click **Finish** arrow.

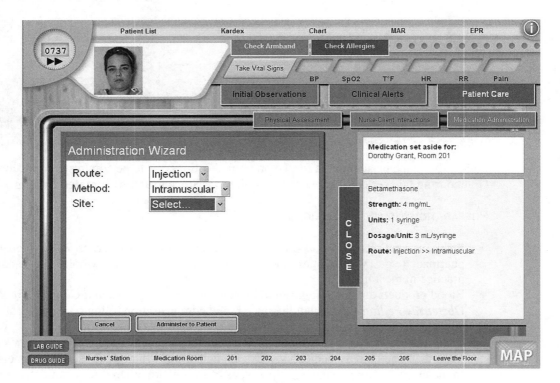

Your selections are recorded by a tracking system and evaluated on a Medication Scorecard stored under Preceptor's Evaluations. This scorecard can be viewed, printed, and given to your instructor. To access the Preceptor's Evaluations, click on **Leave the Floor**. When the Floor Menu appears, select **Look at Your Preceptor's Evaluation**. Then click on **Medication Scorecard** inside the box with Dorothy Grant's name (see example on the following page).

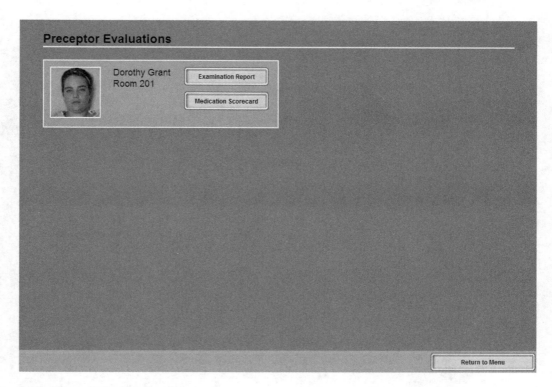

■ MEDICATION SCORECARD

- First, review Table A. Was betamethasone given correctly? Did you give the other medications as ordered?
- Table B shows you which (if any) medications you gave incorrectly.
- Table C addresses the resources used for Dorothy Grant. Did you access the patient's chart, MAR, EPR, or Kardex as needed to make safe medication administration decisions?
- Did you check the patient's armband to verify her identity? Did you check whether your patient had any known allergies to medications? Were vital signs taken?

When you have finished reviewing the scorecard, click **Return to Evaluations** and then **Return to Menu**.

■ VITAL SIGNS

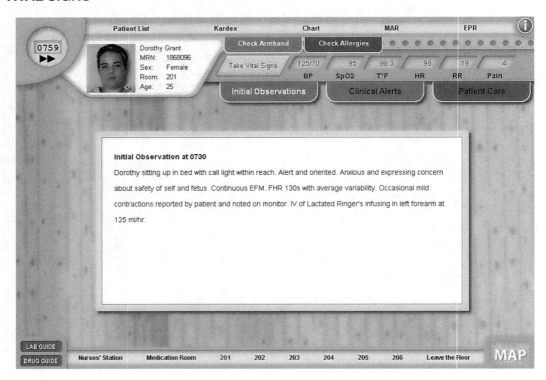

Vital signs, often considered the traditional "signs of life," include body temperature, heart rate, respiratory rate, blood pressure, oxygen saturation of the blood, and pain level.

Inside Dorothy Grant's room, click **Take Vital Signs**. (*Note:* If you are following this detailed tour step by step, you will need to **Restart the Program** from the Floor Menu, sign in again for Period of Care 1, and navigate to Room 201.) Collect vital signs for this patient and record them below. Note the time at which you collected each of these data. (*Remember:* You can take vital signs at any time. The data change over time to reflect the temporal changes you would find in a patient similar to Dorothy Grant.)

Vital Signs	Findings/Time
Blood pressure	
O$_2$ saturation	
Temperature	
Heart rate	
Respiratory rate	
Pain rating	

After you are done, click on the **EPR** icon located in the tool bar at the top of the screen. Your username and password are automatically provided. Click on **Login** to enter the EPR. To access Dorothy Grant's records, click on the down arrow next to Patient and choose her room number, **201**. Select **Vital Signs** as the category. Next, in the empty time column on the far right, record the vital signs data you just collected in the patient's room. If you need help with this process, refer to the Electronic Patient Record (EPR) section of the Quick Tour. Now compare these findings with the data you collected earlier for this patient's vital signs. Use these earlier findings to establish a baseline for each of the vital signs.

    a.   Are any of the data you collected significantly different from the baseline for a particular vital sign?

        Circle One: Yes   No

    b.   If "Yes," which data are different?

■ PHYSICAL ASSESSMENT

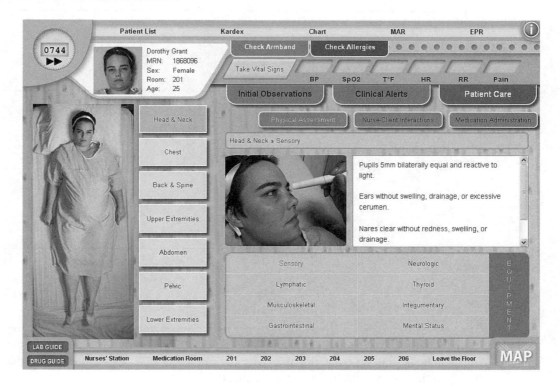

After you have finished examining the EPR for vital signs, click **Exit EPR** to return to Room 201. Click **Patient Care** and then **Physical Assessment**. Think about the information you received in the report at the beginning of this shift, as well as what you may have learned about this patient from the chart. Based on this, what area(s) of examination should you pay most attention to at this time? Is there any equipment you should be monitoring? Conduct a physical assessment of the body areas and systems that you consider priorities for Dorothy Grant. For example, select **Head & Neck**; then click on and assess **Sensory** and **Lymphatic**. Complete any other assessment(s) you think are necessary at this time. In the following table, record the data you collected during this examination.

Area of Examination	Findings
Head & Neck Sensory	
Head & Neck Lymphatic	

After you have finished collecting these data, return to the EPR. Compare the data that were already in the record with those you just collected.

a. Are any of the data you collected significantly different from the baselines for this patient?

Circle One: Yes   No

b. If "Yes," which data are different?

■ NURSE-CLIENT INTERACTIONS

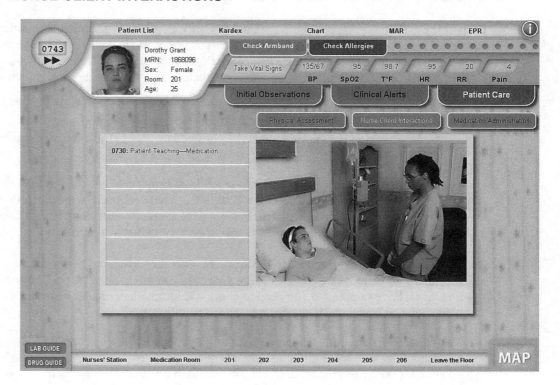

Click on **Patient Care** from inside Dorothy Grant's room (201). Now click on **Nurse-Client Interactions** to access a short video titled **Patient Teaching—Medication**, which is available for viewing at or after 0730 (based on the virtual clock in the upper left corner of your screen; see *Note* below). To begin the video, click on the white arrow next to its title. You will observe a nurse communicating with Dorothy Grant. There are many variations of nursing practice, some exemplifying "best" practice and some not. Note whether the nurse in this interaction displays professional behavior and compassionate care. Are her words congruent with what is going on with the patient? Does this interaction "feel right" to you? If not, how would you handle this situation differently? Explain.

Note: If the video you wish to view is not listed, this means you have not yet reached the correct virtual time to view that video. Check the virtual clock; you may return to access the video once its designated time has occurred—as long as you do so within the same period of care. Or you can click on the fast-forward icon within the virtual clock to advance the time by 2-minute intervals. You will then need to click again on **Patient Care** and **Nurse-Client Interactions** to refresh the screen.

At least one Nurse-Client Interactions video is available during each period of care. Viewing these videos can help you learn more about what is occurring with a patient at a certain time and also prompt you to discern between nurse communications that are ideal and those that need improvement. Compassionate care and the ability to communicate clearly are essential components of delivering quality nursing care, and it is during your clinical time that you will begin to refine these skills.

■ COLLECTING AND EVALUATING DATA

Each of the activities you perform in the Patient Care environment generates a significant amount of assessment data. Remember that after you collect data, you can record your findings in the EPR. You can also review the EPR, patient's chart, videos, and MAR at any time. You will get plenty of practice collecting and then evaluating data in context of the patient's course.

Now, here's an important question for you:

> Did the previous sequence of exercises provide the most efficient way to assess Dorothy Grant?

For example, you went to the patient's room to get vital signs, then back to the EPR to enter data and compare your findings with extant data. Next, you went back to the patient's room to do a physical examination, then again back to the EPR to enter and review data. If this back-and-forth process of data collection and recording seemed inefficient, remember the following:

- Plan all of your nursing activities to maximize efficiency, while at the same time optimizing the quality of patient care. (Think about what data you might need before performing certain tasks. For example, do you need to check a heart rate before administering a cardiac medication or check an IV site before starting an infusion?)

- You collect a tremendous amount of data when you work with a patient. Very few people can accurately remember all these data for more than a few minutes. Develop efficient assessment skills, and record data as soon as possible after collecting them.

- Assessment data are only the starting point for the nursing process.

Make a clear distinction between these first exercises and how you actually provide nursing care. These initial exercises were designed to involve you actively in the use of different software components. This workbook focuses on sensible practices for implementing the nursing process in ways that ensure the highest-quality care of patients.

Most important, remember that a human being changes through time, and that these changes include both the physical and psychosocial facets of a person as a living organism. Think about this for a moment. Some patients may change physically in a very short time (a patient with emerging myocardial infarction) or more slowly (a patient with a chronic illness). Patients' overall physical and psychosocial conditions may improve or deteriorate. They may have effective coping skills and familial support, or they may feel alone and full of despair. In fact, each individual is a complex mix of physical and psychosocial elements, and at least some of these elements usually change through time.

Thus it is crucial that you *DO NOT* think of the nursing process as a simple one-time, five-step procedure consisting of assessment, nursing diagnosis, planning, implementation, and evaluation. Rather, the nursing process should be utilized as a creative and systematic approach to delivering nursing care. Furthermore, because all living organisms are constantly changing, we must apply the nursing process over and over. Each time we follow the nursing process for an individual patient, we refine our understanding of that patient's physical and psychosocial conditions based on collection and analysis of many different types of data. *Virtual Clinical Excursions—Obstetrics-Pediatrics* will help you develop both the creativity and the systematic approach needed to become a nurse who is equipped to deliver the highest-quality care to all patients.

REDUCING MEDICATION ERRORS

Earlier in the detailed tour, you learned the basic steps of medication preparation and administration. The following simulations will allow you to practice those skills further—with an increased emphasis on reducing medication errors by using the Medication Scorecard to evaluate your work.

Sign in to work on the Obstetrics Floor at Pacific View Regional Hospital for Period of Care 1. (*Note:* If you are already working with another patient or during another period of care, click on **Leave the Floor** and then **Restart the Program**; then sign in.)

From the Patient List, select Dorothy Grant. Then click on **Go to Nurses' Station**. Complete the following steps to prepare and administer medications to Dorothy Grant.

- Click on **Medication Room** on the tool bar at the bottom of your screen.
- Click on **MAR** and then on tab **201** to determine medications that have been ordered for Dorothy Grant. (*Note:* You may click on **Review MAR** at any time to verify the correct medication order. Always remember to check the patient name on the MAR to make sure you have the correct patient's record. You must click on the correct room number tab within the MAR.) Click on **Return to Medication Room** after reviewing the correct MAR.
- Click on **Unit Dosage** (or on the Unit Dosage cabinet); from the close-up view, click on drawer **201**.
- Select the medications you would like to administer. After each selection, click **Put Medication on Tray**. When you are finished selecting medications, click **Close Drawer** and then **View Medication Room**.
- Click **Automated System** (or on the Automated System unit itself). Click **Login**.
- On the next screen, specify the correct patient and drawer location.
- Select the medication you would like to administer and click **Put Medication on Tray**. Repeat this process if you wish to administer other medications from the Automated System.
- When you are finished, click **Close Drawer** and **View Medication Room**.
- From the Medication Room, click **Preparation** (or on the preparation tray).
- From the list of medications on your tray, highlight the correct medication to administer and click **Prepare**.
- This activates the Preparation Wizard. Supply any requested information; then click **Next**.
- Now select the correct patient to receive this medication and click **Finish**.
- Repeat the previous three steps until all medications that you want to administer are prepared.
- You can click on **Review Your Medications** and then on **Return to Medication Room** when ready. Once you are back in the Medication Room, go directly to Dorothy Grant's room by clicking on **201** at the bottom of the screen.
- Inside the patient's room, administer the medication, utilizing the six rights of medication administration. After you have collected the appropriate assessment data and are ready for administration, click **Patient Care** and then **Medication Administration**. Verify that the correct patient and medication(s) appear in the left-hand window. Highlight the first medication you wish to administer; then click the down arrow next to Select. From the drop-down menu, select **Administer** and complete the Administration Wizard by providing any information requested. When the Wizard stops asking for information, click **Administer to Patient**. Specify **Yes** when asked whether this administration should be recorded in the MAR. Finally, click **Finish**.

■ **SELF-EVALUATION**

Now let's see how you did during your medication administration!

• Click on **Leave the Floor** at the bottom of your screen. From the Floor Menu, select **Look at Your Preceptor's Evaluation**. Then click **Medication Scorecard**.

The following exercises will help you identify medication errors, investigate possible reasons for these errors, and reduce or prevent medication errors in the future.

1. Start by examining Table A. These are the medications you should have given to Dorothy Grant during this period of care. If each of the medications in Table A has a ✓ by it, then you made no errors. Congratulations!

If any medication has an X by it, then you made one or more medication errors.

Compare Tables A and B to determine which of the following types of errors you made: Wrong Dose, Wrong Route/Method/Site, or Wrong Time. Follow these steps:
  a. Find medications in Table A that were given incorrectly.
  b. Now see if those same medications are in Table B, which shows what you actually administered to Dorothy Grant.
  c. Comparing Tables A and B, match the Strength, Dose, Route/Method/Site, and Time for each medication you administered incorrectly.
  d. Then, using the form below, list the medications given incorrectly and mark the errors you made for each medication.

Medication	Strength	Dosage	Route	Method	Site	Time
	❑	❑	❑	❑	❑	❑
	❑	❑	❑	❑	❑	❑
	❑	❑	❑	❑	❑	❑
	❑	❑	❑	❑	❑	❑

2. To help you reduce future medication errors, consider the following list of possible reasons for errors.

• Did not check drug against MAR for correct medication, correct dose, correct patient, correct route, correct time, correct documentation.
• Did not check drug dose against MAR three times.
• Did not open the unit dose package in the patient's room.
• Did not correctly identify the patient using two identifiers.
• Did not administer the drug on time.
• Did not verify patient allergies.
• Did not check the patient's current condition or vital sign parameters.
• Did not consider why the patient would be receiving this drug.
• Did not question why the drug was in the patient's drawer.
• Did not check the physician's order and/or check with the pharmacist when there was a question about the drug or dose.
• Did not verify that no adverse effects had occurred from a previous dose.

Based on the list of possibilities you just reviewed, determine how you made each error and record the reason in the form below:

Medication	Reason for Error

3. Look again at Table B. Are there medications listed that are not in Table A? If so, you gave a medication to Dorothy Grant that she should not have received. Complete the following exercises to help you understand how such an error might have been made.

   a. Perhaps you gave a medication that was on Dorothy Grant's MAR for this period of care, without recognizing that a change had occurred in the patient's condition, which should have caused you to reconsider. Review patient records as necessary and complete the following form:

Medication	Possible Reasons Not to Give This Medication

   b. Another possibility is that you gave Dorothy Grant a medication that should have been given at a different time. Check her MAR and complete the form below to determine whether you made a Wrong Time error:

Medication	Given to Dorothy Grant at What Time	Should Have Been Given at What Time

c. Maybe you gave another patient's medication to Dorothy Grant. In this case, you made a Wrong Patient error. Check the MARs of other patients and use the form below to determine whether you made this type of error:

Medication	Given to Dorothy Grant	Should Have Been Given to

4. The Medication Scorecard provides some other interesting sources of information. For example, if there is a medication selected for Dorothy Grant but it was not given to her, there will be an X by that medication in Table A, but it will not appear in Table B. In that case, you might have given this medication to some other patient, which is another type of Wrong Patient error. To investigate further, look at Table D, which lists the medications you gave to other patients. See whether you can find any medications ordered for Dorothy Grant that were given to another patient by mistake. However, before you make any decisions, be sure to cross-check the MAR for other patients because the same medication may have been ordered for multiple patients. Use the following form to record your findings:

Medication	Should Have Been Given to Dorothy Grant	Given by Mistake to

5. Now take some time to review the medication exercises you just completed. Use the form below to create an overall analysis of what you have learned. Once again, record each of the medication errors you made, including the type of each error. Then, for each error you made, indicate specifically what you would do differently to prevent this type of error from occurring again.

Medication	Type of Error	Error Prevention Tactic

Submit this form to your instructor if required as a graded assignment, or simply use these exercises to improve your understanding of medication errors and how to reduce them.

Name: _____   Date: _____

KEY ICONS

The following icons are used throughout this workbook to help you quickly identify particular activities and assignments:

 Indicates a reading assignment—tells you which textbook chapter(s) you should read before starting each lesson

 Indicates a writing activity

 Marks the beginning of an interactive virtual hospital activity—signals you to return to your *Virtual Clinical Excursions* simulation

 Indicates additional virtual hospital activity instructions

 Indicates questions and activities that require you to consult your textbook

 Indicates the approximate time required to complete an exercise

LESSON **1**

Community Care: The Family and Culture

🕶 **Reading Assignment:** Community Care: The Family and Culture (Chapter 2)

Patients: Dorothy Grant, Room 201
Stacey Crider, Room 202
Kelly Brady, Room 203
Maggie Gardner, Room 204
Gabriela Valenzuela, Room 205
Laura Wilson, Room 206

Objectives:

- Assess and plan care for a patient from a specific culture.
- Explore how your background influences the care that you give to patients who have differing experiences in regard to community, family, or culture.
- Discuss the various types of families, communities, and cultures represented by each of the patients.

Exercise 1

 Virtual Hospital Activity

 15 minutes

Review pages 17-18 in your textbook and complete the following exercise regarding family types.

Read question 1 before starting this period of care. Fill in the table as you review each patient's chart.

- Sign in to work at Pacific View Regional Hospital on the Obstetrics Floor for Period of Care 1. (*Note*: If you are already in the virtual hospital from a previous exercise, click on **Leave the Floor** and then **Restart the Program** to get to the sign-in window.)
- From the Patient List, select all the patients to review.
- Click on **Go to Nurses' Station** and then on **Chart**.
- Click on Dorothy Grant's chart (**201**) to begin.
- Click on the **Admissions** tab and find the patient's marital status.
- Once you have completed the column for Dorothy Grant in the table below, click on **Return to Nurses' Station** and review Stacey Crider's chart (**202**). Repeat this sequence until you have completed question 1.

1. Under each patient's name below, place an X to indicate that patient's type of family.

	Dorothy Grant	Stacey Crider	Kelly Brady	Maggie Gardner	Gabriela Valenzuela	Laura Wilson
Nuclear						
Multigenerational						
Married-parent						
Single-parent						
Married-blended						

2. Using what you learned in your chart review combined with the information in your textbook, describe the type of family that Gabriela Valenzuela has.

3. Based on the information provided in your textbook, what type of family do you have? Describe how your family fits the description of the family type that you have chosen.

Exercise 2

Virtual Hospital Activity

 25 minutes

- Sign in to work at Pacific View Regional Hospital on the Obstetrics Floor for Period of Care 1. (*Note*: If you are already in the virtual hospital from a previous exercise, click on **Leave the Floor** and then **Restart the Program** to get to the sign-in window.)
- From the Patient List, select Stacey Crider and Maggie Gardner.
- Click on **Go to Nurses' Station**.
- Click on **Chart** and then on **202**.
- Click on **Nursing Admission**.
- Review Stacey Crider's Nursing Admission. (*Hint*: See the Role Relationships section.)

1. Identify a nursing diagnosis that would be appropriate for Stacey Crider and her family.

→ • Click on **Return to Nurses' Station** and open Maggie Gardner's chart by clicking on **Chart** and then on **204**.
- Click on **Nursing Admission**.
- Review Maggie Gardner's Nursing Admission. (*Hint*: See the Health Promotion section.)

2. What alternative therapy/complementary therapy does Maggie Gardner use to relieve stomach trouble?

 3. According to the chart on page 26 in the textbook, what other condition(s) do members of Maggie Gardner's cultural group tend to self-treat during pregnancy?

Maggie Gardner and her husband are very religious. According to the textbook, most members of the African-American culture have strong feelings about family, community, and religion. With this information in mind, complete the following activity and questions.

 • Click on **Return to Nurses' Station**.
• Click on Room **204** at the bottom of the screen.
• Click on **Patient Care** and then **Nurse-Client Interactions**.
• Select and view the video titled **0730: Communicating Empathy**. (*Note:* Check the virtual clock to see whether enough time has elapsed. You can use the fast-forward feature to advance the time by 2-minute intervals if the video is not yet available. Then click on **Patient Care** and **Nurse-Client Interactions** to refresh the screen.)

4. What does Maggie Gardner's husband verbalize during this interaction that would correlate with the African-American population's deep sense of religion?

5. Based on interacting with patients in the hospital where you have worked, describe your experience(s) with caring for someone of a different culture. What are some of the ideals that are different from your own? What barriers have you experienced to your care?

6. How comfortable are you with caring for patients from a different culture? Do you find yourself feeling judgmental or attempting to change others? What can you do to learn more about other cultures?

7. What resources are available at your hospital or within your community to enhance your ability to care for a culturally diverse population?

To further explore Jim and Maggie Gardner's spiritual perspective of this event, return to the patient's chart.

- Click on **Chart** and then on **204**.
- Click on **Consultations**.
- Review the Pastoral Care Spiritual Assessment and the Pastoral Consultation. (*Hint:* Be sure to scroll down to read all the pages in this section.)

8. What does Maggie Gardner "blame" her miscarriages on?

9. Based on your review, what is Maggie Gardner's perception of God?

10. Based on your review of Maggie Gardner's chart during this exercise, what is one underlying theme that you see in the Consultations, Nursing Admission, and History and Physical in regard to religion and this patient's perception of her situation?

Exercise 3

 Virtual Hospital Activity

 15 minutes

 Just as there are different types of families, there are also various vulnerable populations of women within every community. To gain a better understanding of this, read pages 32-34 of the textbook.

Read question 1 before starting this period of care. Fill in the table as you review each patient's chart.

- Sign in to work at Pacific View Regional Hospital on the Obstetrics Floor for Period of Care 1. (*Note*: If you are already in the virtual hospital from a previous exercise, click on **Leave the Floor** and then **Restart the Program** to get to the sign-in window.)
- From the Patient List, select all six patients.
- Click on **Go to Nurses' Station** and then on **Chart**.
- Select Dorothy Grant's chart (**201**) to begin.
- Click on **Nursing Admission**. (*Hint*: The first four pages of this section will provide information regarding the patient's population.)
- You may also click on the **History and Physical** for information to complete the table below.
- Once you have completed Dorothy Grant's column in question 1, click on **Return to Nurses' Station**. Repeat the above steps for each patient.

1. Under each patient's name in the table below, place an X next to each description that applies.

	Dorothy Grant	Stacey Crider	Kelly Brady	Maggie Gardner	Gabriela Valenzuela	Laura Wilson
Adolescent						
Minority						
Older						
Migrant						
Homeless						
Immigrant						

2. Laura Wilson is a member of one of the most medically underserved groups. What are two lifestyle choices she has made that represent high-risk behaviors common in this group?

3. According to information in the textbook, Dorothy Grant could be classified as homeless. As a woman, what are two contributing factors to homelessness?

4. According to the textbook, women who are in racial and ethnic minorities experience a

   disproportionate burden of _____, _____, and

   _____ death.

5. According to the textbook, minority women with underlying health conditions have an

   increased risk for _____.

6. What has your experience been with caring for vulnerable populations?

7. Based on the information found in the textbook, will you change the way you care for these patients in the future? If so, how? In your community, what resources are available for women who are affected by the issues discussed in this exercise?

Exercise 4

 Clinical Preparation: Writing Activity

 15 minutes

 Read pages 32-38 in your textbook.

1. List two possible nursing diagnoses for perinatal home health care patients?

2. What are the six areas included in the psychosocial assessment?

3. What should you do if you identify neglect or abuse within the home while conducting a home visit?

LESSON 2

Substance Abuse/ Violence Against Women

 Reading Assignment: Assessment and Health Promotion (Chapter 3)

Patients: Dorothy Grant, Room 201
                 Laura Wilson, Room 206

Objectives:

- Assess and plan care for a substance-abusing woman with a term pregnancy.
- Discuss the statistics related to intimate partner violence (IPV).
- List characteristics of battered women.
- Explore the myths and facts regarding IPV.
- Identify the nurse's role in regard to battered women or those involved in IPV.

Exercise 1

 Virtual Hospital Activity

🕐 20 minutes

- Sign in to work at Pacific View Regional Hospital on the Obstetrics Floor for Period of Care 2. (*Note*: If you are already in the virtual hospital from a previous exercise, click on **Leave the Floor** and then **Restart the Program** to get to the sign-in window.)
- From the Patient List, select Laura Wilson.
- Click on **Go to Nurses' Station**.
- Click on **Chart** and then on **206**.
- Click on **Nursing Admission**.

1. Complete the table by documenting Laura Wilson's use of alcohol and recreational drugs, based on your review of the Nursing Admission.

Substance	Reported Use
Tobacco	
Alcohol	
Marijuana	
Crack cocaine	

 Read about tobacco, alcohol, marijuana, and cocaine in the Substance Use and Abuse section on pages 53-56 in your textbook.

2. For each pregnancy-related risk listed in the table below, place an X under the substance(s) thought to be associated with that risk.

Pregnancy-Related Risk	Tobacco	Alcohol	Marijuana	Cocaine
Miscarriage				
Placental perfusion abnormalities				
Preterm labor/birth				
Abruptio placentae				
Fetal alcohol syndrome (FAS)				
Fetal alcohol effects (FAE)				
Stillbirth				
Fetal anomalies				
Low birth weight or fetal growth restriction				
Mental retardation/ developmental problems				
Sudden infant death syndrome (SIDS)				

- Click on **Return to Nurses' Station**.
- Click on **206** at the bottom of the screen.
- Click on **Patient Care** and then on **Nurse-Client Interactions**.
- Select and view the video titled **1115: Teaching—Effects of Drug Use**. (*Note:* Check the virtual clock to see whether enough time has elapsed. You can use the fast-forward feature to advance the time by 2-minute intervals if the video is not yet available. Then click on **Patient Care** and **Nurse-Client Interactions** to refresh the screen.)

3. Does Laura Wilson consider herself to be addicted? Support your answer with comments from the video.

4. How does Laura Wilson think her drug use will affect her baby?

5. According to the nurse in the video, how might Laura Wilson's drug use affect the baby?

6. Assume that you are the nurse caring for Laura Wilson today. Which interventions to deal with Laura Wilson's drug use would be most appropriate at this time?

_____   Talk with Laura Wilson in a manner that conveys caring and concern.

_____   Urge Laura Wilson to begin a drug treatment program today.

_____   Explain to Laura Wilson that she may lose custody of her baby if her drug use continues.

_____   Involve other members of the health care team in Laura Wilson's care.

7. Explain your choice(s) in question 6.

Exercise 2

 Virtual Hospital Activity

15 minutes

 Review the information on pages 60-63 in your textbook.

   1. Match the statistics on the right to the descriptions of abuse on the left.

      _____ Number of women who are victims of IPV in the United States

      _____ Estimates of number of women experiencing IPV during pregnancy

      _____ Number of women who are victimized by stalkers

      a. 5.2 million women/year

      b. 4% to 8%; may be as much as 20%

      c. 1 in 4 women

➜ • Sign in to work at Pacific View Regional Hospital on the Obstetrics Floor for Period of Care 1. (*Note*: If you are already in the virtual hospital from a previous exercise, click on **Leave the Floor** and then **Restart the Program** to get to the sign-in window.)

   • From the Patient List, select Dorothy Grant.

   • Click on **Go to Nurses' Station**.

   • Click on **Chart** and then on **201**.

   • Click on **Nursing Admission**.

 In reading about Dorothy Grant's perspective on the abusive relationship she has experienced, compare and contrast this information with content regarding intimate partner violence found in the textbook.

   2. What is the reality of Dorothy Grant's situation? How does that correlate with the textbook reading?

➜ • Click on **Return to Nurses' Station**.

   • Click on Room **201** at the bottom of the screen.

   • Click on **Patient Care** and then **Nurse-Client Interactions**.

   • Select and view the video titled **0810: Monitoring/Patient Support**. (*Note:* Check the virtual clock to see whether enough time has elapsed. You can use the fast-forward feature to advance the time by 2-minute intervals if the video is not yet available. Then click on **Patient Care** and **Nurse-Client Interactions** to refresh the screen.)

3. In the video interaction, what does Dorothy Grant verbalize that she should do to help prevent the violence?

4. In the video, what are the patient's concerns at the moment?

→ • Click on **Chart** and then on **201**.
  • Review the **History and Physical** and the **Nursing Admission** as needed to answer question 5.

5. Battered women have certain characteristics. For each characteristic listed below and on the next page, discuss how Dorothy Grant compares. Base your answers on what you have learned about the patient so far in your chart review and in the video interaction at 0810.

Financially dependent

Few resources/support systems

Blame themselves for what has taken place

State that they are not "good enough"

Bonding occurs out of fear and helplessness

Low self-esteem

History of domestic violence in their family

Fear societal rejection

Strong nurturing, yielding personality

Tolerate control from others easily

Attempt to avoid arousing anger in the abuser

Experience deliberate/repeated physical or sexual assault

Exercise 3

Virtual Hospital Activity

10 minutes

- Sign in to work at Pacific View Regional Hospital on the Obstetrics Floor for Period of Care 3. (*Note*: If you are already in the virtual hospital from a previous exercise, click on **Leave the Floor** and then **Restart the Program** to get to the sign-in window.)
- From the Patient List, select Dorothy Grant.
- Click on **Go to Nurses' Station**.
- Click on **Chart** and then on **201**.
- Click on **Consultations** and review the Psychiatric Consult and the Social Work Consult.

Review the information regarding the myths and facts about intimate partner violence on page 61 (Table 3-2) in the textbook. Based on that information and your review of Dorothy Grant's chart, answer the following:

1. Dorothy Grant stays in the relationship because of _____ and _____.

2. The percentage of women who are battered during pregnancy is _____.

3. Based on the information provided, in what phase of the abuse cycle is Dorothy Grant?

4. According to the consults, Dorothy Grant has several options. What are some of the options that the social worker and psychiatric heath care provider can offer her or assist her with?

5. Battering often escalates or begins during pregnancy.
   a. True
   b. False

6. Dorothy Grant's husband blames her for the pregnancy.
   a. True
   b. False

7. Dorothy Grant stays in the relationship because she likes to be beaten and deliberately provokes the attacks on occasion.
   a. True
   b. False

Exercise 4

Virtual Hospital Activity

15 minutes

- Sign in to work at Pacific View Regional Hospital on the Obstetrics Floor for Period of Care 4. (*Note*: If you are already in the virtual hospital from a previous exercise, click on **Leave the Floor** and then **Restart the Program** to get to the sign-in window.)
- From the Nurses' Station, click on **Kardex** and then on tab **201** to review Dorothy Grant's record. (*Remember:* You are not able to visit patients or administer medications during Period of Care 4. You are able to review patient records only.)

1. What action was initiated on Wednesday to protect Dorothy Grant from her husband?

2. What care plan diagnoses are appropriate for this patient's current life situation?

3. What other disciplines have been contacted or consulted that will ensure continuity of care for Dorothy Grant as it relates to her abuse?

 Review pages 61-63 in your textbook before answering the following questions.

4. As a nurse caring for Dorothy Grant, what is your responsibility for reporting IPV?

5. What are the reporting requirements of the state in which you practice?

6. What are the resources available in your area for women who have experienced intimate partner violence?

LESSON 3

Maternal and Fetal Nutrition; Assessment of Risk Factors

 Reading Assignment: Maternal and Fetal Nutrition (Chapter 9)

Assessment of High Risk Pregnancy (Chapter 10): Psychologic Considerations Related to High Risk Pregnancy; Ultrasonography; Biophysical Profile

High Risk Perinatal Care: Preexisting Conditions (Chapter 11): Anemia

Patients: Kelly Brady, Room 203
Maggie Gardner, Room 204
Laura Wilson, Room 206

Objectives:

- Identify appropriate interventions for maintaining adequate maternal and fetal nutrition.
- Differentiate among the varying types of assessment techniques that can be used with both low- and high-risk pregnant patients.
- Identify various methods of testing that can be used in high-risk pregnancies.

Exercise 1

 Virtual Hospital Activity

 15 minutes

Review information on pages 249-251 in the textbook.

1. A high-risk pregnancy is one in which the life or health of _____ or

_____ is jeopardized by _____ coincidental with or unique to the pregnancy.

- Sign in to work at Pacific View Regional Hospital on the Obstetrics Floor for Period of Care 3. (*Note:* If you are already in the virtual hospital from a previous exercise, click on **Leave the Floor** and then **Restart the Program** to get to the sign-in window.)
- From the Patient List, select Kelly Brady (Room 203), Maggie Gardner (Room 204), and Laura Wilson (Room 206).
- Click on **Go to Nurses' Station**.

- Click on **Chart**.
- For each of these three patients, open the chart, click on **History and Physical**, and review the report.

2. After reviewing the History and Physical, list the things that place each of these patients at risk during their pregnancy.

Kelly Brady

Maggie Gardner

Laura Wilson

Review information regarding ultrasounds on pages 252-256 in the textbook.

3. List three things that ultrasounds are used for in the first trimester and then in the second/third trimester.

First trimester

Second/third trimester

4. What are two forms of ultrasound? When are they used?

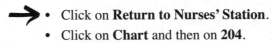 • Click on **Return to Nurses' Station**.
- Click on **Chart** and then on **204**.
- Click on **Diagnostic Reports**.

5. What type of ultrasound is Maggie Gardner having?

6. Based on the ultrasound findings, how large is her baby?

7. List three abnormalities found on the ultrasound in regard to the placenta.

8. What is the impression from Maggie Gardner's ultrasound in terms of the fetus and the placenta?

9. What are the recommendations regarding follow-up?

Exercise 2

Virtual Hospital Activity

15 minutes

 Biophysical profile is another very important assessment tool used with patients who are experiencing a high-risk pregnancy. Review information regarding biophysical profiles on pages 256-257 in the textbook.

1. What are the five items that are assessed on a biophysical profile?

2. When an abnormal _____ and _____ are encountered,

_____ is warranted.

3. The biophysical profile is a reliable indicator of _____.

4. The normal score on a biophysical profile is _____.

→ • Sign in to work at Pacific View Regional Hospital on the Obstetrics Floor for Period of Care 3. (*Note*: If you are already in the virtual hospital from a previous exercise, click on **Leave the Floor** and then **Restart the Program** to get to the sign-in window.)
  • From the Patient List, select Kelly Brady (Room 203).
  • Click on **Go to Nurses' Station**.
  • Click on **Chart** and then on **203**.
  • Click on **Diagnostic Reports** and review.

5. What is the estimated gestational age of Kelly Brady's fetus?

6. What is the amniotic fluid index as indicated on the report?

7. How does this correlate with the normal index as listed in the textbook?

8. What is the score on the biophysical profile?

9. Based on the information you have learned through your review of the textbook, what does this score indicate?

Exercise 3

 Virtual Hospital Activity

 15 minutes

- Sign in to work at Pacific View Regional Hospital on the Obstetrics Floor for Period of Care 1. (*Note*: If you are already in the virtual hospital from a previous exercise, click on **Leave the Floor** and then **Restart the Program** to get to the sign-in window.)
- From the Patient List, select Maggie Gardner (Room 204).
- Click on **Go to Nurses' Station**.
- Click on **Chart** and then on **204**.
- Click on **Laboratory Reports**.

 Review pages 290-292 in the textbook for information regarding anemia.

1. What were Maggie Gardner's hemoglobin and hematocrit levels on admission?

 • Click on **History and Physical**.

2. What puts Maggie Gardner at a greater risk for developing anemia than the average pregnancy patient? (*Hint*: Review the Genetic Screening section of her History and Physical.)

3. What complications may women with anemia or sickle cell anemia experience in pregnancy?

4. What is a normal hematocrit level for women who are pregnant?

5. How is anemia defined through a woman's hemoglobin and hematocrit levels?

6. What assessments need to be performed by the nurse at each visit specifically related to an anemia diagnosis?

Review Chapter 9 regarding nutrition, iron supplementation, and dietary sources.

7. According to Table 9-1 in the textbook, what are some good sources of iron that you could instruct Maggie Gardner to add to her diet?

8. Maggie Gardner is not on iron supplementation at this time; however, list three things that you could teach her about iron supplementation. (*Hint*: See page 245 of your textbook.)

9. A woman who consumes 200 mg of caffeine per day during pregnancy may be at an

   increased risk for _____ and may contribute to _____.

LESSON 4

Reproductive System Concerns

 Reading Assignment: Reproductive System Concerns (Chapter 4):
Human Immunodeficiency Virus; Bacterial Vaginosis

Patients: Stacey Crider, Room 202
Gabriela Valenzuela, Room 205
Laura Wilson, Room 206

Objectives:

- Assess and plan care for a pregnant woman with bacterial vaginosis.
- Explain the importance of prophylactic Group B streptococcus treatment.
- Identify risk factors for acquiring HIV infection.
- Prioritize information to be included in patient teaching related to HIV infection.

Exercise 1

 Virtual Hospital Activity

15 minutes

- Sign in to work at Pacific View Regional Hospital on the Obstetrics Floor for Period of Care 1. (*Note*: If you are already in the virtual hospital from a previous exercise, click on **Leave the Floor** and then **Restart the Program** to get to the sign-in window.)
- From the Patient List, select Stacey Crider (Room 202).
- Click on **Go to Nurses' Station**.
- Click on **Chart** and then on **202**.
- Click on **History and Physical**.

1. In the table below, describe Stacey Crider's vaginal discharge based on her diagnosis on admission. How does it compare with the description of bacterial vaginosis found on page 97 in the textbook?

	Stacey Crider's Discharge	Textbook Description
Appearance		
Amount		
Odor		

2. How is bacterial vaginosis diagnosed?

3. Which medication is recommended for treating bacterial vaginosis during pregnancy?

→ • Now click on **Physician's Orders** in the chart.
   • Scroll down to the admitting physician's orders on Tuesday at 0630.

4. What are Stacey Crider's admission diagnoses?

5. Explain how Stacey Crider's admission diagnoses are likely to be related.

6. Which medication did Stacey Crider's physician order to treat her bacterial vaginosis?

7. Assume that Stacey Crider is discharged home on day 4 of the prescribed treatment with the medication you identified in question 6. What specific information about this medication should she be taught? (*Hint*: Check page 97 in the textbook.)

 • Click on **Return to Nurses' Station**.

Exercise 2

 Virtual Hospital Activity

 15 minutes

• Sign in to work at Pacific View Regional Hospital on the Obstetrics Floor for Period of Care 1. (*Note*: If you are already in the virtual hospital from a previous exercise, click on **Leave the Floor** and then **Restart the Program** to get to the sign-in window.)
• From the Patient List, select Gabriela Valenzuela (Room 205).
• Click on **Go to Nurses' Station**.
• Click on **Chart** and then on **205**.
• Click on **History and Physical** and scroll to the plan at the end of this document.

1. What is the medical plan of care for Gabriela Valenzuela?

2. Is Gabriela Valenzuela known to be positive for Group B streptococcus (GBS)?

 Read about Group B streptococcus on pages 98-99 in your textbook; then answer questions 3 through 6.

3. List risk factors for neonatal GBS infection. Which risk factor applies to Gabriela Valenzuela?

4. Since pregnant women with GBS in the vagina are almost always asymptomatic, why does Gabriela Valenzuela need to be treated for this organism?

 • Click on **Physician's Orders**.
   • Scroll to the admission orders written Tuesday at 2100.

5. What medication/dosage/frequency will Gabriela Valenzuela receive for Group B strep prophylaxis?

6. How does this order compare with the treatment regimen recommended in your textbook?

 • Click on **Return to Nurses' Station**.

Exercise 3

 Virtual Hospital Activity

 35 minutes

• Sign in to work at Pacific View Regional Hospital on the Obstetrics Floor for Period of Care 1. (*Note*: If you are already in the virtual hospital from a previous exercise, click on **Leave the Floor** and then **Restart the Program** to get to the sign-in window.)
• From the Patient List, select Laura Wilson (Room 206).
• Click on **Go to Nurses' Station**.
• Click on **Chart** and then on **206**.
• Click on **Nursing Admission**.

1. What risk factors for acquiring an STI are identified on Laura Wilson's Nursing Admission form?

2. List specific risk factors for acquiring HIV infection. (*Hint:* See page 85 in the textbook.) Place an asterisk next to the risk factors that are present in Laura Wilson's history.

3. What did the admitting nurse document about Laura Wilson's knowledge and acceptance of her HIV diagnosis?

 • Click on **Return to Nurses' Station** and then on **206** at the bottom of the screen.
 • Click on **Patient Care** and then **Nurse-Client Interactions**.
 • Select and view the video titled **0800: Teaching—HIV in Pregnancy**. (*Note:* Check the virtual clock to see whether enough time has elapsed. You can use the fast-forward feature to advance the time by 2-minute intervals if the video is not yet available. Then click on **Patient Care** and **Nurse-Client Interactions** to refresh the screen.)

4. Does Laura Wilson appear to be fully aware of the implications of HIV infection? State the rationale for your answer.

5. What coping mechanism is Laura Wilson exhibiting in the video interaction?

 • Click on **Chart** and then on **206**.
 • Click on **Nursing Admission**.

6. Laura Wilson needs education on all of the following topics. Which would you choose to teach her about at this time?

_____ Safer sex

_____ Medication side effects and importance of compliance

_____ Need for medical follow-up and medication for the baby

_____ Impact of HIV on birth plans

7. Give a rationale for your answer to question 6.

Common Reproductive Concerns, Infertility, and Contraception

 Reading Assignment: Assessment and Health Promotion (Chapter 3)
Reproductive System Concerns (Chapter 4): Amenorrhea
Infertility, Contraception, and Abortion (Chapter 5): Infertility;
Contraception

Patients: Stacey Crider, Room 202
Kelly Brady, Room 203
Maggie Gardner, Room 204
Gabriela Valenzuela, Room 205
Laura Wilson, Room 206

Objectives:

- Identify reproductive issues that can occur.
- Differentiate among the various types of contraception options.
- Identify various methods of testing and treatment options that can be used for couples experiencing infertility.

Exercise 1

 Virtual Hospital Activity

 10 minutes

Review information on pages 46-48 in your textbook.

1. What is a normal length for a menstrual cycle?

2. What are the criteria required to diagnose an individual with amenorrhea? Differentiate between primary and secondary amenorrhea.

• Sign in to work at Pacific View Regional Hospital on the Obstetrics Floor for Period of Care 1. (*Note*: If you are already in the virtual hospital from a previous exercise, click on **Leave the Floor** and then **Restart the Program** to get to the sign-in window.)
   • From the Patient List, select Stacey Crider (Room 202).
   • Click on **Go to Nurses' Station**.
   • Click on **Chart** and then on **202**.
   • Click on **History and Physical**.
   • Review the patient's gynecologic history. (*Hint:* See the bottom of page 1.)

3. Does Stacey Crider meet the textbook criteria for amenorrhea?

4. What is her history?

5. List three things that can cause amenorrhea.

Exercise 2

 Virtual Hospital Activity

 20 minutes

 Review pages 110-120 in your textbook.

1. _____% of the reproductive age population has a problem with infertility.

2. A fertile couple has a _____% chance of conception in each ovulatory cycle.

Maggie Gardner is 41 years old. Let's consider some of the options she had while attempting to get pregnant.

3. List factors that affect female fertility. (*Hint:* Refer to Box 5-1.)

4. List factors that affect male fertility. (*Hint:* Refer to Box 5-2.)

- Sign in to work at Pacific View Regional Hospital on the Obstetrics Floor for Period of Care 1. (*Note*: If you are already in the virtual hospital from a previous exercise, click on **Leave the Floor** and then **Restart the Program** to get to the sign-in window.)
- From the Patient List, select Maggie Gardner (Room 204).
- Click on **Go to Nurses' Station**.
- Click on **Chart** and then on **204**.
- Review the **History and Physical**.

5. Maggie Gardner was married _____ years prior to conceiving the first time.

6. Based on the textbook reading, which of the following would Maggie Gardner have been diagnosed with if she had chosen to get treatment after a year of attempting to get pregnant?
   a. Primary infertility
   b. Secondary infertility

 Review pages 112-115 in your textbook to answer the following questions.

7. What four tests can be completed on a female patient to determine the causes of infertility?

8. What two tests can be completed on a male patient to determine the causes of infertility?

9. What two tests are used to assess ovarian reserve?

10. What medical and nonmedical treatments are available to assist an infertile couple in conceiving?

11. What methods did Maggie Gardner and her husband use to assist in getting pregnant? (*Hint*: Review the OB history in the History and Physical.)

Exercise 3

Virtual Hospital Activity

 20 minutes

 Review pages 120-139 in the textbook.

1. What is contraception?

2. Providing contraception doesn't necessarily mean preventing _____.

 • Sign in to work at Pacific View Regional Hospital on the Obstetrics Floor for Period of Care 1. (*Note*: If you are already in the virtual hospital from a previous exercise, click on **Leave the Floor** and then **Restart the Program** to get to the sign-in window.)
   • From the Patient List, select Kelly Brady (Room 203), Gabriela Valenzuela (Room 205), and Laura Wilson (Room 206).
   • Click on **Go to Nurses' Station**.
   • Click on **Chart** and then on **203** for Kelly Brady's chart.
   • Review the **History and Physical**.
   • Click on **Go to Nurses' Station** and repeat the previous two steps for Gabriela Valenzuela and Laura Wilson.

3. Identify the birth control method each woman was using prior to her current pregnancy.

Kelly Brady

Gabriela Valenzuela

Laura Wilson

4. Only _____ methods provide protection against STIs.

5. Gabriela Valenzuela is Catholic. Which method would be appropriate for the nurse to discuss with her?

6. What does this method rely on?

7. Kelly Brady desires to use oral contraceptives while breastfeeding to prevent pregnancy. Which type of oral contraception is appropriate for her to use? Why?

8. Laura Wilson is HIV-positive. What is the most appropriate form of birth control for her? Why?

High Risk Perinatal Care: Gestational Diabetes Mellitus

 Reading Assignment: High Risk Perinatal Care: Preexisting Conditions (Chapter 11): Diabetes Mellitus; Gestational Diabetes Mellitus

Patient: Stacey Crider, Room 202

Objectives:

- Identify appropriate interventions for controlling hyperglycemia in a patient with gestational diabetes mellitus (GDM).
- Correctly administer insulin to a patient with GDM.
- Plan and evaluate essential patient teaching for a patient with GDM.

Exercise 1

 Virtual Hospital Activity

30 minutes

- Sign in to work at Pacific View Regional Hospital on the Obstetrics Floor for Period of Care 2. (*Note*: If you are already in the virtual hospital from a previous exercise, click on **Leave the Floor** and then **Restart the Program** to get to the sign-in window.)
- From the Patient List, select Stacey Crider (Room 202).
- Click on **Go to Nurses' Station**.
- Click on **Chart** and then on **202**.
- Click on **History and Physical**.

1. When was Stacey Crider's GDM diagnosed? How has it been managed thus far?

2. Read about risk factors for GDM on page 279 in your textbook. List these factors below.

→ • Search for evidence of the risk factors for GDM in Stacey Crider in the **History and Physical** and **Admissions** sections of her chart.

3. Which risk factors for GDM are present in Stacey Crider?

4. What does Stacey Crider's physician suspect is the cause of her poorly controlled blood glucose levels? (*Hint*: See Impression at the end of the History and Physical.)

→ • Click on **Physician's Orders**.

5. Look at Stacey Crider's admission orders. Write down the orders that are related to GDM.

6. Why did Stacey Crider's physician order a hemoglobin A_{1C} test as part of her admission labs? (*Hint*: See page 273 in your textbook.) What is the desired lab value level?

On admission, Stacey Crider is in preterm labor. This was treated with magnesium sulfate tocolysis. She was also given a course of betamethasone.

 • Click on **Return to Nurses' Station**.
• Click on the **Drug** icon in the lower left corner of the screen.
• Scroll down the drug list and click on **betamethasone**.

7. How might betamethasone affect Stacey Crider's GDM?

 • Click on **Return to Nurses' Station**.
• Click on **Chart** and then on **202**.
• Click on **Physician's Notes**.
• Scroll to the note for Tuesday at 0700.

8. How does Stacey Crider's physician plan to deal with these potential medication effects?

Stacey Crider's other admission diagnosis is bacterial vaginosis (BV).

• Click on **Return to Nurses' Station**.
• Click on **202** at the bottom of the screen.
• Click on **Patient Care** and then on **Nurse-Client Interactions**.
• Select and view the video titled **1115: Teaching—Diet, Infection**. (*Note:* Check the virtual clock to see whether enough time has elapsed. You can use the fast-forward feature to advance the time by 2-minute intervals if the video is not yet available. Then click on **Patient Care** and **Nurse-Client Interactions** to refresh the screen.)

9. What is the relationship between Stacey Crider's bacterial vaginosis infection and her GDM?

Exercise 2

Virtual Hospital Activity

20 minutes

- Sign in to work at Pacific View Regional Hospital on the Obstetrics Floor for Period of Care 1. (*Note*: If you are already in the virtual hospital from a previous exercise, click on **Leave the Floor** and then **Restart the Program** to get to the sign-in window.)
- From the Patient List, select Stacey Crider (Room 202).
- Click on **Go to Nurses' Station**.

Stacey Crider needs her insulin so that she can eat breakfast. Recall that she receives lispro insulin prior to each meal and NPH insulin at bedtime. Read about the differences in these two types of insulin in your textbook.

1. Based on your textbook reading, complete the table below. (*Note*: NPH is considered an intermediate-acting insulin.)

Type of Insulin	Onset of Action	Peak	Duration
Lispro			
Intermediate-acting			

- Click on **EPR** and then on **Login**.
- Click on **202** in the Patient drop-down menu. Click on **Vital Signs** in the Category drop-down menu.
- Look at the vital sign assessment documented on Wednesday at 0700.

2. What is Stacey Crider's blood glucose?

- Click on **Exit EPR**.
- Click on **MAR**.
- Click on tab **202**.

3. What is Stacey Crider's prescribed lispro insulin dosage?

- Click on **Return to Nurses' Station**.
- Click on **Chart** and then on **202**.
- Click on **Physician's Orders**.
- Scroll to the orders for Tuesday at 1900.

4. How much insulin should Stacey Crider receive? Why?

- Click on **Return to Nurses' Station**.
- Click on **Medication Room** at the bottom of the screen.
- Click on **Unit Dosage**.
- Click on drawer **202**.
- Click on **Insulin Lispro**.
- Click on **Put Medication on Tray**.
- Click on **Close Drawer** at the bottom of the screen.
- Click on **View Medication Room**.
- Click on **Preparation**.
- Click on **Prepare** and follow the prompts to complete preparation of Stacey Crider's lispro insulin dose.
- Click on **Return to Medication Room**.

You are almost ready to give Stacey Crider's insulin injection. However, before you do . . .

5. Considering the rapid onset of action of lispro insulin, what else should you check before giving Stacey Crider her injection?

Now you're ready!

- Click on Room **202**.
- Click on **Check Armband**.
- Click on **Patient Care**.
- Click on **Medication Administration**.
- **Insulin Lispro** should be listed on the left side of your screen. Click on the down arrow next to **Select** and choose **Administer**.
- Follow the prompts to administer Stacey Crider's insulin injection. Click on **Administer to Patient**.
- Indicate **Yes** to document the injection in the MAR. Click on **Finish**.
- Click on **Leave the Floor**.
- Click on **Look at Your Preceptor's Evaluation**.
- Click on **Medication Scorecard**. How did you do?
- Click on **Return to Evaluations** and then on **Return to Menu**.

Exercise 3

 Virtual Hospital Activity

 20 minutes

- Sign in to work at Pacific View Regional Hospital on the Obstetrics Floor for Period of Care 3. (*Note*: If you are already in the virtual hospital from a previous exercise, click on **Leave the Floor** and then **Restart the Program** to get to the sign-in window.)
- From the Patient List, select Stacey Crider (Room 202).
- Click on **Go to Nurses' Station**.
- Click on **Chart** and then on **202**.
- Click on **Patient Education**.

Stacey Crider will likely be discharged home soon. Review her Patient Education record to determine her learning needs in relation to GDM.

1. List the educational goals for Stacey Crider regarding GDM.

 Read the section on Antepartum Care on pages 279-281 in your textbook.

2. Which of Stacey Crider's educational goals would apply to all women with GDM?

3. Which of Stacey Crider's educational goals would *not* apply to all women with GDM? Support your answer.

➜ • Click on **Nurse's Notes** and scroll to the note for 0600 Wednesday.

4. How did the nurse describe Stacey Crider's ability to give her own insulin injection at that time?

➜ • Click again on **Patient Education**.

5. What teaching has already been done with this patient on Wednesday in regard to GDM?

➜ • Click on **Nurse's Notes** and scroll to the note for 1200 Wednesday.

6. Do you think today's initial teaching on insulin administration was effective? Support your answer using objective documentation from the nurse's note.

Use the information you have obtained from the Patient Education form and the Nurse's Notes to answer the following questions.

7. Stacey Crider needs to know all of the following information. Which topic(s) would you choose to work on with her during this period of care?

_____   Verbalize appropriate food choices and portions.

_____   Demonstrate good technique when administering insulin.

_____   Demonstrate good technique with self-monitoring of blood glucose.

_____   Recognize hyper- and hypoglycemia and how to treat each.

8. Give a rationale for your answer to question 7.

9. Which topic do you think Stacey Crider would choose to work on during this period of care?

_____ Verbalize appropriate food choices and portions.

_____ Demonstrate good technique when administering insulin.

_____ Demonstrate good technique with self-monitoring of blood glucose.

_____ Recognize hyper- and hypoglycemia and how to treat each.

10. Give a rationale for your answer to question 9.

Read the section on Postpartum Care on page 282 in your textbook. Stacey Crider has a significant risk for developing glucose intolerance later in life.

11. What advice would you give Stacey Crider to reduce this risk?

12. After delivery, what medical follow-up would you advise for Stacey Crider?

13. Could Stacey Crider's GDM affect her baby after birth? Explain.

LESSON 7

High Risk Perinatal Care: Cardiac Disorders, Lupus

 Reading Assignment: High Risk Perinatal Care: Preexisting Conditions (Chapter 11): Cardiovascular Disorders; Systemic Lupus Erythematosus (SLE)

Patients: Maggie Gardner, Room 204
Gabriela Valenzuela, Room 205

Objectives:

- Identify appropriate interventions for managing selected medical-surgical problems in pregnancy.
- Plan and evaluate essential patient education during the acute phase of diagnosis.

Exercise 1

 Virtual Hospital Activity

 10 minutes

- Sign in to work at Pacific View Regional Hospital on the Obstetrics Floor for Period of Care 1. (*Note*: If you are already in the virtual hospital from a previous exercise, click on **Leave the Floor** and then **Restart the Program** to get to the sign-in window.)
- From the Patient List, select Gabriela Valenzuela (Room 205).
- Click on **Go to Nurses' Station**.
- Click on **Chart** and then on **205**.
- Click on **History and Physical**.

Review material regarding cardiac problems during pregnancy on pages 284-286 in the textbook.

85

1. According to the textbook, 0.5%-4% of pregnancies are complicated with heart disease. In the History and Physical for Gabriela Valenzuela, what does the physician note as her cardiac problem?

2. Mitral valve disease is one of the most common causes of cardiac disease in pregnant women.
   a. True
   b. False

3. According to the History and Physical, what cardiac symptoms does Gabriela Valenzuela exhibit now that she is pregnant?

4. Based on your textbook reading, why do pregnant women with cardiac disorders have problems during their pregnancy?

5. What abnormal assessment finding is noted in the History and Physical that would be associated with Gabriela Valenzuela's cardiac disorder?

Exercise 2

 Virtual Hospital Activity

 20 minutes

 Autoimmune disorders encompass a wide variety of disorders that can be disruptive to the pregnancy process. Maggie Gardner has been admitted to rule out lupus. The following activities will explore the various aspects of this autoimmune disorder. First, review pages 296-297 in your textbook regarding systemic lupus erythematosus (SLE).

* Sign in to work at Pacific View Regional Hospital on the Obstetrics Floor for Period of Care 1. (*Note*: If you are already in the virtual hospital from a previous exercise, click on **Leave the Floor** and then **Restart the Program** to get to the sign-in window.)
* From the Patient List, select Maggie Gardner (Room 204).
* Click on **Go to Nurses' Station**.
* Click on **Chart** and then on **204**.
* Click on **History and Physical**.

1. Based on Maggie Gardner's History and Physical, what information would correlate with a diagnosis of SLE?

2. According to the textbook, pregnant women with SLE have additional maternal risks and tend to experience increased rates of several conditions or complications. Identify at least three of these complications or conditions that occur at increased rates in pregnant women with SLE.

 • Click on **Return to Nurses' Station**.
• Click on Room **204** at the bottom of the screen.
• Click on **Patient Care**.
• Click on **Physical Assessment**.
• Click on the various body areas (yellow boxes) and system subcategories (green boxes) to perform a head-to-toe assessment of Maggie Gardner.

3. Based on your head-to-toe assessment, list four abnormal findings that are related to Maggie Gardner's diagnosis.

 • Click on **Chart** and then on **204**.
• Click on **Patient Education**.

4. Based on your physical assessment, the information from the Patient Education section of the chart, and the fact that this is a new diagnosis for the patient, list three areas of teaching that need to be completed with this patient.

Exercise 3

Virtual Hospital Activity

35 minutes

- Sign in to work at Pacific View Regional Hospital on the Obstetrics Floor for Period of Care 3. (*Note*: If you are already in the virtual hospital from a previous exercise, click on **Leave the Floor** and then **Restart the Program** to get to the sign-in window.)
- From the Patient List, select Maggie Gardner (Room 204).
- Click on **Go to Nurses' Station**.
- Click on **Chart** and then on **204**.
- Click on the **Consultations** tab.
- Review the Rheumatology Consult.

1. List four findings that the rheumatologist notes in her impressions associated with a diagnosis of SLE.

2. What is the rheumatologist's plan regarding laboratory/diagnostics to gain a definitive diagnosis?

3. According to the Rheumatology Consult, what is the plan regarding medications (immediate need)?

→ • Click on **Diagnostic Reports**.

    4. Maggie Gardner had an ultrasound done prior to the consult with the rheumatologist. What were the findings as they relate to SLE? What were the follow-up recommendations? (*Hint*: See Impressions section.)

→ • Click on **Return to Nurses' Station**.
  • Click on the **Drug** icon in the lower left corner of the screen.
  • Find the Drug Guide profile of prednisone. (*Hint:* You can type the drug name in the Search box or scroll through the alphabetic list of drugs at the top of the screen.)

    5. What does Maggie Gardner need to be taught regarding this medication?

→ • Click on **Return to Nurses' Station**.
  • Click on Room **204** at the bottom of the screen.
  • Click on **Patient Care** and then **Nurse-Client Interactions**.
  • Select and view the video titled **1530: Disease Management**. (*Note:* Check the virtual clock to see whether enough time has elapsed. You can use the fast-forward feature to advance the time by 2-minute intervals if the video is not yet available. Then click on **Patient Care** and **Nurse-Client Interactions** to refresh the screen.)

6. During this video clip, the nurse provides Maggie Gardner with information regarding her disease. What two things does the nurse note that are important aspects of the patient's disease management during pregnancy?

7. What medication ordered by the rheumatologist will assist in the blood flow to the placenta? How?

8. What key component does the nurse identify for Maggie Gardner that will assist in maintaining a healthy pregnancy?

9. What excuse does Maggie Gardner give for not keeping previous doctors' appointments? (*Hint:* This information is found in the Nursing Admission in the chart.)

Exercise 4

 Virtual Hospital Activity

 15 minutes

- Sign in to work at Pacific View Regional Hospital on the Obstetrics Floor for Period of Care 4. (*Note:* If you are already in the virtual hospital from a previous exercise, click on **Leave the Floor** and then **Restart the Program** to get to the sign-in window.)
- From the Nurses' Station, click on **Chart**. (*Remember:* You are not able to visit patients or administer medications during Period of Care 4. You are able to review patients' records only.)
- Click on **204** to open Maggie Gardner's chart.
- Click on **Laboratory Reports**.

1. The results are now available for the following laboratory tests that were ordered in Period of Care 2. What are the findings?

Laboratory Test	Result
C4	
CH50	
RPR	
ANA titer	
Anticardiolipin	
Anti-sm; Anti-DNA; Anti–SSA	
Anti-SSB	
Anti-RVV; Antiphospholipid	

➤ • Click on **Consultations** and review the Rheumatology Consult.

2. The lab findings you recorded in question 1 are definitive for the diagnosis of SLE. According to the textbook and the Rheumatology Consult, what is the plan to manage this disease once the baby is delivered?

➤ • Click on **Nurse's Notes.**

3. By Period of Care 4, Maggie Gardner has been provided with education regarding various aspects of her disease process, testing, and hospital procedures. Based on your review of the Nurse's Notes for Wednesday, what has she been specifically taught? Include the time each instruction took place.

4. Using correct NANDA nursing diagnosis terminology, write three possible nursing diagnoses for Maggie Gardner.

5. SLE requires long-term management because patients will experience remissions and exacerbations. What step did the rheumatologist take with Maggie Gardner to begin the long-term relationship that will be required to ensure a healthy outcome?

6. What is Maggie Gardner's risk for having an exacerbation during her pregnancy or during the postpartum period?

7. What is the typical recommendation regarding multiple future pregnancies for women who have SLE? Why?

LESSON 8

High Risk Perinatal Care: Severe Preeclampsia

 Reading Assignment: High Risk Perinatal Care: Gestational Conditions
(Chapter 12): Hypertension in Pregnancy

Patient: Kelly Brady, Room 203

Objectives:

- Assess and identify signs and symptoms present in the patient with severe preeclampsia.
- Explain how common signs and symptoms present in the patient with severe preeclampsia relate to the underlying pathophysiology of this disease.
- Identify the patient who has developed HELLP syndrome.
- Describe routine nursing care for the patient with severe preeclampsia who is receiving magnesium sulfate.

Exercise 1

 Virtual Hospital Activity

🕐 20 minutes

- Sign in to work at Pacific View Regional Hospital on the Obstetrics Floor for Period of Care 3. (*Note*: If you are already in the virtual hospital from a previous exercise, click on **Leave the Floor** and then **Restart the Program** to get to the sign-in window.)
- From the Patient List, select Kelly Brady (Room 203).
- Click on **Go to Nurses' Station**.
- Click on **Chart** and then on **203**.
- Click on **History and Physical**.

1. What was Kelly Brady's admission diagnosis?

2. Use the History and Physical and page 304 in your textbook to complete the table below.

Sign/Symptom	Mild Preeclampsia	Severe Preeclampsia	Kelly Brady on Admission
Blood pressure			
Proteinuria			
Headache			
Irritability or changes in affect			
Visual problems			
Epigastric pain			

➤ • Click on **Physician's Orders** and find the admitting physician's orders on Tuesday at 1030.

3. What tests/procedures did Kelly Brady's physician order to confirm the diagnosis of severe preeclampsia?

➤ • Click on **Physician's Notes**.
  • Scroll to the note for Wednesday 0730.

4. What subjective and objective data are recorded here that would support the diagnosis of severe preeclampsia?

Kelly Brady's 24-hour urine collection was completed and sent to the lab at 1230.

➤ • Click on **Laboratory Reports**.
  • Scroll to find the Wednesday 1230 results.

5. Below, record the results of Kelly Brady's 24-hour urine collection.

6. Now list all the data you have collected during this exercise that confirm Kelly Brady's diagnosis of severe preeclampsia.

Exercise 2

Virtual Hospital Activity

 20 minutes

- Sign in to work at Pacific View Regional Hospital on the Obstetrics Floor for Period of Care 1. (*Note*: If you are already in the virtual hospital from a previous exercise, click on **Leave the Floor** and then **Restart the Program** to get to the sign-in window.)
- From the Patient List, select Kelly Brady (Room 203).
- Click on **Go to Nurses' Station**.
- Click on **203** at the bottom of the screen to go to the patient's room.
- Click on **Take Vital Signs**.

1. Record Kelly Brady's vital signs for 0730 below.

→ • Now click on **Patient Care**. To perform a focused assessment, select the various body areas (yellow boxes) and system subcategories (green boxes) as listed in question 2.

2. Record your findings from the focused assessment of Kelly Brady in the table below.

Assessment Area	Kelly Brady's Findings
Head and Neck Sensory	
Neurologic	
Chest Respiratory	
Abdomen Gastrointestinal	
Lower Extremities Neurologic	

Read pages 304-306 in your textbook, then answer questions 3 and 4.

3. The main pathogenic factor present in a woman with preeclampsia is not an

_____, but _____ as a result of

_____ and _____.
As a result, blood flow to all organs may be diminished.

4. Match each of the signs or symptoms below with the preeclampsia-associated pathology it indicates. (*Note:* Some letters will be used more than once.)

_____ Blurred vision/blind spots   a. Generalized vasoconstriction

_____ Headache   b. Glomerular damage

_____ Epigastric or right upper quadrant c. Retinal arteriolar spasms
   abdominal pain

             d. Hepatic edema/subcapsular hemorrhage

_____ 4+ reflexes/clonus

             e. Increased CNS irritability

_____ Elevated blood pressure

_____ Proteinuria/oliguria

Exercise 3

 Virtual Hospital Activity

 30 minutes

- Sign in to work at Pacific View Regional Hospital on the Obstetrics Floor for Period of Care 3. (*Note*: If you are already in the virtual hospital from a previous exercise, click on **Leave the Floor** and then **Restart the Program** to get to the sign-in window.)
- From the Patient List, select Kelly Brady (Room 203).
- Click on **Go to Nurses' Station**.

 Read about HELLP syndrome on page 306 in your textbook.

1. Why do you think Kelly Brady had blood drawn at 1230 for an AST measurement and a platelet count?

- Click on **Chart** and then on **203**.
- Click on **Laboratory Reports**.
- Scroll to the report for Wednesday 1230 to locate the results of these tests.

 2. Complete the table below based on your review of the Laboratory Reports and your textbook.

Test	Wednesday 1230 Result	Value in HELLP
Platelet count		
AST		

- Click on **Return to Nurses' Station**.
- Click on **Patient List**.
- In the far-right column click on **Get Report** for Kelly Brady.

3. Why has Kelly Brady been transferred to labor and delivery?

4. HELLP syndrome is a _____ diagnosis. Characterized by

_____, _____, and _____.

Many women with HELLP syndrome may have no _____.

5. What type of woman is most likely to develop HELLP syndrome? Which of these characteristics is true of Kelly Brady?

→ • Sign in to work at Pacific View Regional Hospital on the Obstetrics Floor for Period of Care 4. (*Note:* If you are already in the virtual hospital from a previous exercise, click on **Leave the Floor** and then **Restart the Program** to get to the sign-in window.)
   • Click on **Chart** and then on **203**. (*Remember:* You are not able to visit patients or administer medications during Period of Care 4. You are able to review patient records only.)
   • Click on **Physician's Notes**.
   • Scroll to the note for Wednesday 1530.

6. What is the physician's plan of care for Kelly Brady, in light of the HELLP syndrome diagnosis?

Assume that you will be the nurse caring for Kelly Brady after her surgery while she is receiving magnesium sulfate. Read about this medication on pages 310-314 in your textbook and then answer question 7.

7. All of the assessments/interventions listed below are part of routine nursing care for a patient with severe preeclampsia. Place an X beside the activities that are performed specifically to assess for magnesium toxicity.

_____ Measure/record urine output.

_____ Measure proteinuria using urine dipstick.

_____ Monitor liver enzyme levels and platelet count.

_____ Monitor for headache, visual disturbances, and epigastric pain.

_____ Assess for decreased level of consciousness.

_____ Assess DTRs.

_____ Weigh daily to assess for edema.

_____ Monitor vital signs, especially respiratory rate.

_____ Dim room lights and maintain a quiet environment.

High Risk Perinatal Care: Antepartal Hemorrhagic Disorders

 Reading Assignment: High Risk Perinatal Care: Gestational Conditions (Chapter 12):
Premature Separation of Placenta

Patient: Gabriela Valenzuela, Room 205

Objectives:

- Identify appropriate interventions for managing abruptio placentae.
- Differentiate between the symptoms related to an abruptio placentae and those related to a placenta previa.
- Plan and evaluate essential patient education during the acute phase of diagnosis.

Exercise 1

 Virtual Hospital Activity

🕐 45 minutes

- Sign in to work at Pacific View Regional Hospital on the Obstetrics Floor for Period of Care 1. (*Note:* If you are already in the virtual hospital from a previous exercise, click on **Leave the Floor** and then **Restart the Program** to get to the sign-in window.)
- From the Patient List, select Gabriela Valenzuela (Room 205).
- Click on **Go to Nurses' Station**.
- Click on **Chart** and then on **205**.
- Click on **Emergency Department**.

1. What transpired that brought Gabriela Valenzuela to the Emergency Department? How long had she waited to actually come to the ED? What was the deciding factor in her coming to the ED?

 Read about the incidence and etiology of abruptio placentae in your textbook in Box 12-7; pages 329-330.

2. Other than a motor vehicle accident, what could result in or increase the risk for having an abruptio placentae?

3. Differential diagnosis is very important when you are confronted with clinical manifestations that could be evidence of more than one process. Based on Table 12-7 on page 327 of your textbook, compare and contrast abruptio placentae and placenta previa.

Characteristic/Complication	Abruptio Placentae	Placenta Previa
Bleeding		
Shock complication		
Coagulopathy (DIC)		
Uterine tonicity		
Tenderness/pain		
Placenta findings		
Fetal effects		
Gestational or chronic hypertension		

4. Based on your review of the ED Record, what grade of abruption does Gabriela Valenzuela have? Provide supporting documentation from your textbook reading. (*Hint*: Review Table 12-7 on page 327.)

 • Click on **Return to Nurses' Station**.
• Click on **205** at the bottom of the screen to go to the patient's room.
• Click on **Patient Care** and then **Nurse-Client Interactions**.
• Select and view the video titled **0740: Patient Teaching—Fetal Monitoring**. (*Note:* Check the virtual clock to see whether enough time has elapsed. You can use the fast-forward feature to advance the time by 2-minute intervals if the video is not yet available. Then click on **Patient Care** and **Nurse-Client Interactions** to refresh the screen.)

5. Once Gabriela Valenzuela is admitted to the floor, what are her and her husband's concerns? What does the nurse include in her teaching to alleviate those concerns?

Gabriela Valenzuela is at increased risk for early delivery as a result of the abdominal trauma she suffered and subsequent occurrence of a grade 1 abruptio placentae. She is currently manifesting signs and symptoms of early labor. According to the Physician's Orders, she was given a dose of betamethasone and this was to be repeated in 12 hours.

 6. What is the purpose of the administration of betamethasone in this patient's case? (*Hint*: Review information on page 450 of the textbook.)

- Click on **MAR** and review the betamethasone dosage to be given to Gabriela Valenzuela.
- Click on **Return to Room 205**.
- Click on **Medication Room** at the bottom of the screen.
- Click on **Unit Dosage**.
- Click on drawer **205**.
- Click on **Betamethasone** in the upper left corner of the screen.
- Click on **Put Medication on Tray**.
- Click on **Close Drawer** at the bottom of the screen.
- Click on **View Medication Room**.
- Click on **Preparation**.
- Click on **Prepare** and follow the Preparation Wizard's prompts to complete preparation of Gabriela Valenzuela's betamethasone.
- When the Administration Wizard stops asking questions, click **Finish**.
- Click on **Return to Medication Room**.
- Click on **205** at the bottom of the screen to return to the patient's room.
- Click on **Patient Care**.
- Click on **Medication Administration**.
- Click on **Review Your Medications**.
- Click on the tab marked **Prepared**.

7. According to the text box on the right side of your screen, what is the medication name and dosage that you have prepared for Gabriela Valenzuela?

8. How many mg are you giving to Gabriela Valenzuela based on the answer to the previous question? Is this the correct dosage based on the MAR?

- Click on **Return to Room 205**.
- Click on the **Drug** icon in the left-hand corner of the screen.
- To read about betamethasone, either type the drug name in the Search box or scroll through the alphabetic list of medications at the top of the screen.

9. Based on the information provided in the Drug Guide, what is the indication and dosage for pregnant adults?

10. Based on your review of the baseline assessment data in the Drug Guide, what areas need to be assessed in Gabriela Valenzuela's history?

11. Now review the information regarding the administration of this medication. What are three things that need to be taken into consideration when giving this medication in the injection form?

12. What are the six rights of medication administration as they relate to the patient?

You are now ready to complete the medication administration.

- Click on **Return to Room 205**.
- Click on **Check Armband**.
- Within the purple box under the patient's photo, find **Betamethasone**. Click the down arrow next to **Select** and choose **Administer**.
- Follow the Medication Wizard's prompts to administer Gabriela Valenzuela's betamethasone. Click **Yes** when asked whether to document the injection in the MAR.
- When the Wizard stops asking questions, click **Finish**.
- Now click on **Patient Care** and then **Nurse-Client Interactions**.
- Select and view the video titled **0805: Patient Teaching—Abruption**. (*Note:* Check the virtual clock to see whether enough time has elapsed. You can use the fast-forward feature to advance the time by 2-minute intervals if the video is not yet available. Then click on **Patient Care** and **Nurse-Client Interactions** to refresh the screen.)

13. According to the video, what will help increase the oxygen supply to the baby and prevent further separation of the placenta?

- Click on **Leave the Floor**.
- Click on **Look at Your Preceptor's Evaluation**.
- Click on **Medication Scorecard** and review the evaluation. How did you do? (*Hint:* For a quick refresher on reading your Medication Scorecard, see page 22 in the **Getting Started** section of this workbook. For a more detailed tour on preparing and administering medications and interpreting your Scorecard, see pages 26-30 and 36-40.)

Exercise 2

Virtual Hospital Activity

30 minutes

- Sign in to work at Pacific View Regional Hospital on the Obstetrics Floor for Period of Care 2. (*Note*: If you are already in the virtual hospital from a previous exercise, click on **Leave the Floor** and then **Restart the Program** to get to the sign-in window.)
- From the Patient List, select Gabriela Valenzuela (Room 205).
- Click on **Go to Nurses' Station**.
- Click on **Chart** and then on **205**.
- Click on **Diagnostic Reports**.

Gabriela Valenzuela had an ultrasound done on Tuesday to determine the source of the bleeding.

1. What were the findings on the ultrasound?

- Click on the **Laboratory Reports**.

2. What were Gabriela Valenzuela's hemoglobin and hematocrit levels on Tuesday? How do these findings compare with Wednesday's report? Has there been a significant change?

3. According to the textbook information, the hematocrit level needs to be maintained at

_____. (*Hint:* See pages 290-292 in the textbook.)

Review management on page 330 in the textbook.

4. What clinical manifestations would indicate suspected abruptio placentae in the condition of either the patient or the fetus?

 • Click on **Return to Nurses' Station**.
 • Click on **EPR**.
 • Click on **Login**.
 • Select **205** from the drop-down list as the patient's room and **Vital Signs** as the category.
 • Using the blue right and left arrows, scroll to review the vital sign findings over the last 12 hours.

5. From 0000 Wednesday until 1200 Wednesday, would you consider Gabriela Valenzuela's condition stable or unstable? State the rationale for your answer.

 • Click on **Exit EPR**.
 • Click on **205** at the bottom of the screen.
 • Click on **Patient Care** and then **Nurse-Client Interactions**.
 • Select and view the video titled **1140: Intervention—Bleeding, Comfort**. (*Note:* Check the virtual clock to see whether enough time has elapsed. You can use the fast-forward feature to advance the time by 2-minute intervals if the video is not yet available. Then click on **Patient Care** and **Nurse-Client Interactions** to refresh the screen.)

6. What happened that elicited this interaction? (*Hint*: Review the Nurse's Notes for Wednesday 1140.)

7. What actions did the nurse take during the interaction?

Exercise 3

Virtual Hospital Activity

15 minutes

- Sign in to work at Pacific View Regional Hospital on the Obstetrics Floor for Period of Care 3. (*Note:* If you are already in the virtual hospital from a previous exercise, click on **Leave the Floor** and then **Restart the Program** to get to the sign-in window.)
- From the Patient List, select Gabriela Valenzuela (Room 205).
- Click on **Go to Nurses' Station**.
- Click on **Kardex** and then on tab **205**.

1. What problem areas have been identified by the nurse related to Gabriela Valenzuela's diagnosis?

2. What is the focus of the outcomes related to the above-mentioned problems?

3. Using correct NANDA nursing diagnosis terminology, list four possible nursing diagnoses appropriate for Gabriela Valenzuela at this time.

→ • Click on **Return to Nurses' Station**.
  • Click on **Chart** and then on **205**.
  • Click on **Patient Education**.

4. According to the Patient Education sheet in Gabriela Valenzuela's chart, what are the educational goals related to the patient's diagnosis?

→ • Click on **Nurse's Notes**.

5. What education has been completed by the nurses through Period of Care 3? Include the times and topics discussed.

6. What are some barriers to learning that the nurse may confront with this patient?

7. How can the nurse overcome each of these?

LESSON 10

Pain Management

 Reading Assignment: Pain Management (Chapter 14)

Patients: Kelly Brady, Room 203
Gabriela Valenzuela, Room 205
Laura Wilson, Room 206

Objectives:

- Assess and identify factors that influence pain perception.
- Describe selected nonpharmacologic and pharmacologic measures for pain management during labor and birth.

Exercise 1

 Virtual Hospital Activity

 45 minutes

- Sign in to work at Pacific View Regional Hospital on the Obstetrics Floor for Period of Care 1. (*Note*: If you are already in the virtual hospital from a previous exercise, click on **Leave the Floor** and then **Restart the Program** to get to the sign-in window.)
- From the Patient List, select Laura Wilson (Room 206).
- Click on **Get Report**.

1. What is Laura Wilson's condition when you assume care for her, according to the change-of-shift report?

→ • Click on **Go to Nurses' Station**.
- Click on Room **206** at the bottom of the screen.
- Read the **Initial Observations**.

2. What is your impression of Laura Wilson's condition?

- Click on **Patient Care** and then **Nurse-Client Interactions**.
- Select and view the video titled **0730: Patient Assessment**. (*Note:* Check the virtual clock to see whether enough time has elapsed. You can use the fast-forward feature to advance the time by 2-minute intervals if the video is not yet available. Then click on **Patient Care** and **Nurse-Client Interactions** to refresh the screen.)

3. What is Laura Wilson's assessment of her current condition? How does this compare with the information you received from the shift report and the Initial Observations summary?

- Click on **Chart** and then on **206**.
- Click on **Nursing Admission**.

4. List Laura Wilson's admission diagnoses. (*Hint:* See page 1 of the Nursing Admission form.)

5. What is your perception of Laura Wilson's behavior? What data did you collect during this exercise that led you to this perception?

6. Think about the following questions and then discuss your ideas with your classmates: Do your personal values and beliefs contribute to your perception of Laura Wilson's behavior? If so, how? What nursing interventions might help to overcome your personal biases when dealing with Laura Wilson?

 Read the section on Factors Influencing Pain Response on pages 357-359 in your textbook.

 Continue reviewing Laura Wilson's **Nursing Admission** form as needed to answer question 7.

7. Each woman's pain during childbirth is unique and is influenced by a variety of factors. For each factor listed below and on the next page, explain how that factor influences pain perception (in the middle column). Then, in the right column, list data from Laura Wilson's Nursing Admission that support how that factor might relate to her particular pain perception.

Factor	Typical Effect on Pain Perception	Laura Wilson's Supporting Data
Anxiety		

Factor	Typical Effect on Pain Perception	Laura Wilson's Supporting Data
Previous experience		
Religion/Culture		
Support		

→ • Click on **Return to Room 206**.

Exercise 2

Virtual Hospital Activity

45 minutes

• Sign in to work at Pacific View Regional Hospital on the Obstetrics Floor for Period of Care 2. (*Note*: If you are already in the virtual hospital from a previous exercise, click on **Leave the Floor** and then **Restart the Program** to get to the sign-in window.)

• From the Patient List, select Gabriela Valenzuela (Room 205).

Read the sections on Nonpharmacologic Pain Management in your textbook (pages 359-365).

1. Touch and massage have been an _____ part of the traditional care process for women in labor. Head, hand, back, and foot massage may be very effective in

   _____ and _____.

2. Different approaches to childbirth preparation use _____

   to help the woman _____.

   _____ is the technique most associated with prepared childbirth.

   All patterns begin and end with a _____.

➡ • Click on **Get Report**.

3. Is Gabriela Valenzuela in labor at this time? Give a rationale for your answer.

➡ • Click **Go to Nurses' Station**.
   • Click on Room **205** at the bottom of the screen.
   • Click on **Patient Care** and then **Nurse-Client Interactions**.
   • Select and view the video titled **1140: Intervention—Bleeding, Comfort**. (*Note:* Check the virtual clock to see whether enough time has elapsed. You can use the fast-forward feature to advance the time by 2-minute intervals if the video is not yet available. Then click on **Patient Care** and **Nurse-Client Interactions** to refresh the screen.)
   • Click on **Chart** and then **205**.
   • Click on **Nurse's Notes**.
   • Scroll to the entry for 1140 on Wednesday.

4. How is Gabriela Valenzuela tolerating labor at this time?

5. What pain interventions does the nurse implement at this time?

 Read the Medication Guide on fentanyl on pages 368-369 in your textbook.

➡ • Click on **Return to Room 205**.

6. What is the action of this drug?

Let's begin the process for preparing and administering Gabriela Valenzuela's fentanyl dose.

- First, click on **Medication Room** at the bottom of the screen.
- Next, click on **MAR** and then on tab **205**.
- Scroll down to the PRN Medication Administration Record for Wednesday.

7. What is the ordered dose of fentanyl?

- Click on **Return to Medication Room**.
- Click on **Automated System**.
- Click on **Login**.
- In box 1, click on **Gabriela Valenzuela, 205**.
- In box 2, click on **Automated System Drawer A-F**.
- Click on **Open Drawer**.
- Click on **Fentanyl citrate**.
- Click on **Put Medication on Tray**.
- Click on **Close Drawer** at the bottom of the screen.
- Click on **View Medication Room**.
- Click on **Preparation**.
- Click on **Prepare** and follow the Preparation Wizard prompts to complete preparation of Gabriela Valenzuela's fentanyl dose. When the Wizard stops requesting information, click **Finish**.
- Click on **Return to Medication Room**.
- Click on **205** at the bottom of the screen to go to the patient's room.

8. What additional assessments must be completed before you give Gabriela Valenzuela's medication?

9. Why is it important to check Gabriela Valenzuela's respirations prior to giving the dose of fentanyl?

10. What safety precautions should be in effect for Gabriela Valenzuela after she receives this dose of fentanyl?

 • Click on **Patient Care** and then **Medication Administration**.
  • Click on **Review Your Medications** and verify the accuracy of your preparation. Click **Return to Room 205**.
  • Next, click the down arrow next to **Select** and choose **Administer**.
  • Follow the Administration Wizard prompts to administer Gabriela Valenzuela's fentanyl dose. (*Note:* Click **Yes** when asked whether to document this administration in the MAR.)
  • When the Wizard stops asking questions, click **Finish**.
  • Still in Gabriela Valenzuela's room, click on **Patient Care** and then **Nurse-Client Interactions**.
  • Select and view the video titled **1155: Evaluation—Comfort Measures**. (*Note:* Check the virtual clock to see whether enough time has elapsed. You can use the fast-forward feature to advance the time by 2-minute intervals if the video is not yet available. Then click on **Patient Care** and **Nurse-Client Interactions** to refresh the screen.)

11. How effective were the interventions you identified in question 5?

12. Gabriela Valenzuela is experiencing _____. _____

    is responsible for the dizziness as well as other side effects, including

    _____, _____, and

    _____.

13. What interventions does the nurse suggest to deal with this problem? List other interventions described in your textbook.

At the end of the 1155 video, Gabriela Valenzuela states that she "doesn't want any needles" in her back. Learn more about this by reading the section on Epidural Analgesia/Anesthesia on pages 374-376 in your textbook.

14. What could you tell Gabriela Valenzuela to help her make an informed decision about anesthesia for labor? Below, list advantages and disadvantages of epidural anesthesia.

Advantages	Disadvantages

Before leaving this period of care, let's see how you did preparing and administering the patient's medication.

- Click on **Leave the Floor**.
- Click on **Look at Your Preceptor's Evaluation**.
- Click on **Medication Scorecard** and review the evaluation. How did you do? (*Hint:* For a quick refresher on reading your Medication Scorecard, see page 22 in the **Getting Started** section of this workbook. For a more detailed tour on preparing and administering medications and interpreting your Scorecard, see pages 26-31 and 36-40.)
- Click on **Return to Evaluations**.
- Click on **Return to Menu**.

Exercise 3

 Virtual Hospital Activity

 20 minutes

 Read the section on General Anesthesia on pages 415-418 in your textbook.

- Sign in to work at Pacific View Regional Hospital on the Obstetrics Floor for Period of Care 4. (*Note:* If you are already in the virtual hospital from a previous exercise, click on **Leave the Floor** and then **Restart the Program** to get to the sign-in window.)
- From the Nurses' Station, click on **Chart** and then on **203** for Kelly Brady's chart. (*Remember:* You are not able to visit patients or administer medications during Period of Care 4. You are able to review patient records only.)
- Click on **Nurse's Notes**.
- Scroll to the entry for 1730 on Wednesday.

1. Why does the anesthesiologist plan to use general anesthesia during Kelly Brady's cesarean section? (*Hint*: Read the section on Contraindications to Epidural Blocks on pages 375-376 in your textbook.)

2. Why is Kelly Brady upset about receiving general anesthesia for her surgery?

 • Click on **Physician's Orders**.
• Review the entry for Wednesday at 1540.

3. What preoperative medications are ordered for Kelly Brady?

 • Click on **Return to Nurses' Station**.
• Click on the **Drug** icon in the lower left corner of your screen to access the Drug Guide.
• Use the Search box or the scroll bar to read about each of the drugs you listed in question 3.

4. All of these medications are given preoperatively to help prevent aspiration pneumonia. Using information from the Drug Guide and from the section on General Anesthesia in your textbook, match each of the medications below with the description of how it specifically works to prevent aspiration pneumonia.

_____ Sodium citrate/citric acid (Bicitra)   a. Decreases the production of gastric acid

_____ Metoclopramide (Reglan)   b. Prevents nausea and vomiting and accelerates gastric emptying

_____ Ranitidine (Zantac)   c. Neutralizes acidic stomach contents

5. During general anesthesia, a short-acting barbiturate is administered to

_____. A muscle relaxer is then given to facilitate

_____. A low concentration of a volatile halogenated agent

may be administered to _____.

6. How would you expect general anesthesia to affect Kelly Brady? Her baby? Why?

Labor and Birth Complications

 Reading Assignment: Labor and Birth Complications (Chapter 17)

Patients: Dorothy Grant, Room 201
Stacey Crider, Room 202
Kelly Brady, Room 203
Gabriela Valenzuela, Room 205

Objectives:

- Assess and identify signs and symptoms present in the patient with preterm labor.
- Describe appropriate nursing care for the patient in preterm labor.
- Develop a birth plan to meet the needs of the preterm infant.

Exercise 1

 Virtual Hospital Activity

20 minutes

- Sign in to work at Pacific View Regional Hospital on the Obstetrics Floor for Period of Care 2. (*Note*: If you are already in the virtual hospital from a previous exercise, click on **Leave the Floor** and then **Restart the Program** to get to the sign-in window.)
- From the Patient List, select Dorothy Grant and Gabriela Valenzuela.
- Click on **Go to Nurses' Station**.
- Click on **Chart** and then on **201** for Dorothy Grant's chart.
- Click on **History and Physical**.

1. Using the information found in the History and Physical section, complete the table below for Dorothy Grant.

Patient	Weeks Gestation	Reason for Admission
Dorothy Grant		

 • Click on **Return to Nurses' Station**.
   • Now click again on **Chart**; this time, select **205** for Gabriela Valenzuela's chart.
   • Click on **History and Physical**.

2. Using the information found in the History and Physical section, complete the table below for Gabriela Valenzuela.

Patient	Weeks Gestation	Reason for Admission
Gabriela Valenzuela		

 • Click on **Return to Nurses' Station**.
   • Click on **201** at the bottom of the screen to go to Dorothy Grant's room.
   • Click on **Patient Care**.
   • Click on **Physical Assessment**.
   • Click on **Pelvic** and then on **Reproductive**.

3. Complete the table below with the results of Dorothy Grant's initial cervical examination.

Patient	Time	Dilation	Effacement	Station
Dorothy Grant				

• Click on **205** at the bottom of the screen to go to Gabriela Valenzuela's room.
   • Click on **Patient Care**.
   • Click on **Physical Assessment**.
   • Click on **Pelvic** and then on **Reproductive**.

4. Record the results of Gabriela Valenzuela's initial cervical examination in the table below.

Patient	Time	Dilation	Effacement	Station
Gabriela Valenzuela				

 Read the section on Early Recognition and Diagnosis of preterm labor on pages 443-445 in your textbook.

5. What criteria are necessary in order to make a diagnosis of preterm labor?

6. As of Wednesday at 0800, would you consider both these patients to be in preterm labor? Give a rationale for your answer.

 Read the section on Suppression of Uterine Activity—Tocolytics on pages 446-450 in your textbook to answer the following questions.

7. Would you recommend tocolytic therapy for Gabriela Valenzuela? Support your answer.

8. Match each of the medications below with the description of how it works as a tocolytic agent. (*Hint:* Letters may be used more than once.)

_____ Magnesium sulfate

_____ Nifedipine (Procardia)

_____ Ritodrine (Yutopar)

_____ Terbutaline (Brethine)

_____ Indomethacin (Indocin)

a. Inhibits calcium from entering smooth muscle cells, thus relaxing uterine contractions

b. Relaxes uterine smooth muscle as a result of stimulation of beta$_2$ receptors on uterine smooth muscle

c. Exact mechanism unclear, but promotes relaxation of smooth muscles

d. Suppresses preterm labor by blocking the production of prostaglandins

Exercise 2

 Virtual Hospital Activity

 30 minutes

- Sign in to work at Pacific View Regional Hospital on the Obstetrics Floor for Period of Care 1. (*Note:* If you are already in the virtual hospital from a previous exercise, click on **Leave the Floor** and then **Restart the Program** to get to the sign-in window.)
- From the Patient List, select Stacey Crider (Room 202).
- Click on **Get Report**.

Stacey Crider was admitted yesterday in preterm labor and placed on magnesium sulfate. Her other admission diagnoses were bacterial vaginosis and gestational diabetes with poorly controlled blood glucose levels.

1. What is Stacey Crider's current status in regard to preterm labor?

 • Click on **Go to Nurses' Station**.
- Click on **Chart** and then on **202**.
- Click on **Physician's Orders**.
- Scroll to the orders for Wednesday at 0715.

2. Which of these orders relate specifically to Stacey Crider's diagnosis of preterm labor?

• Scroll to the orders for Wednesday at 0730.

3. What medication changes are ordered?

 Read about terbutaline and nifedipine in the Tocolytic Therapy for Preterm Labor Medication Guide (pages 447-450) in your textbook.

4. Why do you think Stacey Crider's physician changed his orders so quickly?

 • Click on **Return to Nurses' Station**.
• Click on **202** at the bottom of the screen.
• Inside the patient's room, click on **Take Vital Signs**.

5. What are Stacey Crider's current vital signs?

Temperature

Heart rate

Respiratory rate

Blood pressure

 6. Which of these parameters provides the most important information you would need prior to giving Stacey Crider's nifedipine dose? Why? (*Hint*: Read about nifedipine on pages 449-450 in your textbook.)

Like Dorothy Grant and Kelly Brady, Stacey Crider is also receiving betamethasone.

 Read about Promotion of Fetal Lung Maturity in your textbook on page 450; then answer the following questions.

7. Why are all three of these patients receiving antenatal glucocorticoid therapy?

8. What other benefits does this class of medication seem to provide for preterm infants?

- Click on **MAR**.
- Click on tab **202**.

9. What is Stacey Crider's prescribed betamethasone dosage?

10. How does this dosage compare with the recommended dosage listed in the Antenatal Glucocorticoid Therapy Medication Guide on page 450 of your textbook?

- Click on **Return to Room 202**.
- Click on **Medication Room**.
- Click on **Unit Dosage**.
- Click on drawer **202**.
- Click on **Betamethasone**.
- Click on **Put Medication on Tray**.
- Click on **Close Drawer** at the bottom of the screen.
- Click on **View Medication Room**.
- Click on **Preparation**.
- Click on **Prepare** and follow the Preparation Wizard's prompts to complete preparation of Stacey Crider's betamethasone dose. When the Preparation Wizard has finished asking questions, click **Finish**.
- Click on **Return to Medication Room**.
- Click on **202** to return to Stacey Crider's room.
- Click on **Check Armband**.
- Click on **Check Allergies**.
- Click on **Patient Care**.
- Click on **Medication Administration**.
- Find **Betamethasone** listed on the left side of your screen. To its right, click on the down arrow next to **Select** and choose **Administer**.
- Follow the Administration Wizard's prompts to administer Stacey Crider's betamethasone injection. Indicate **Yes** to document the injection in the MAR.
- When the Preparation Wizard has finished asking questions, click **Finish**.
- Click on **Leave the Floor**.
- Click on **Look at Your Preceptor's Evaluation**.
- Click on **Medication Scorecard**. How did you do?
- Click on **Return to Evaluations**.
- Click on **Return to Menu**.

Exercise 3

Virtual Hospital Activity

30 minutes

- Sign in to work at Pacific View Regional Hospital on the Obstetrics Floor for Period of Care 4. (*Note*: If you are already in the virtual hospital from a previous exercise, click on **Leave the Floor** and then **Restart the Program** to get to the sign-in window.)
- Click on **Chart** and then on **201**. (*Remember:* You are not able to visit patients or administer medications during Period of Care 4. You are able to review patients' records only.)
- Click on **Nurse's Notes**.
- Scroll to the note for Wednesday 1815.

1. What are the findings from Dorothy Grant's cervical examination at this time?

 • Scroll to the note for Wednesday 1840. It states that Dorothy Grant is being prepped for delivery.

2. If you were the nurse caring for Dorothy Grant during delivery, what special preparations would you make to care for the baby immediately after birth?

 • Click on **Return to Nurses' Station**.
- Click again on **Chart**, but this time choose **205** for Gabriela Valenzuela's chart.
- Click on **Physician's Notes**.
- Scroll to the note for Wednesday 0800.

3. What is the anticipated outcome of Gabriela Valenzuela's labor, according to this note?

• Scroll to the notes for Wednesday 1415 and 1455.

4. What preparations have been made during the day for the birth of Gabriela Valenzuela's baby?

 Read the information on cesarean birth found on pages 469-475 in your textbook.

 • Click on **Return to Nurses' Station**.
• Once again, click on **Chart**; select **203** for Kelly Brady's chart.
• Click on **Physician's Notes**.
• Scroll to the note for Wednesday 1530.

Kelly Brady was admitted yesterday with severe preeclampsia at 26 weeks gestation. Her preeclampsia is now worsening.

5. Why does her physician now recommend immediate delivery?

6. What general risks related to cesarean section does Kelly Brady's physician discuss with her?

7. Because of Kelly Brady's early gestational age (26 weeks), her physician anticipates a classical uterine incision. How will this type of incision affect Kelly Brady's birth options in future pregnancies?

• Click on **Physician's Orders**.
 • Scroll to the orders for Wednesday 1540.

8. List the orders to be carried out prior to Kelly Brady's surgery. State the purpose of each.

Order	Purpose

 9. Can you think of other common preoperative procedures? List them below. (*Hint*: Refer to a basic Medical-Surgical textbook for ideas if you need help!)

LESSON 12

The High Risk Newborn: Neonatal Loss

 Reading Assignment: The High Risk Newborn (Chapter 25)

Patient: Maggie Gardner, Room 204

Objectives:

- Identify the various types of loss as they relate to a pregnancy.
- Describe the stages and phases of the grieving process.
- Identify various methods of coping exhibited by patients who have experienced the loss of a newborn.

Exercise 1

 Clinical Preparation: Writing Activity

 10 minutes

Review the information on pages 695-696 in the textbook.

1. The loss of an infant represents _____, _____, or

   _____.

2. At what other times might couples grieve a loss related to pregnancy? (*Hint:* Consider various readings you have completed.)

3. Women experience what type of effects if a pregnancy ends early because of miscarriage?

4. Parents need to be given the opportunity to "parent" the infant in any manner they wish or are able to before and after death.
   a. True
   b. False

5. All women and men who undergo a loss receive the support that they need.
   a. True
   b. False

6. NICU nurses feel helpless and sorrowful. This type of grief must be allowed. Do you agree? Why or why not?

Exercise 2

Virtual Hospital Activity

10 minutes

- Sign in to work at Pacific View Regional Hospital on the Obstetrics Floor for Period of Care 4. (*Note*: If you are already in the virtual hospital from a previous exercise, click on **Leave the Floor** and then **Restart the Program** to get to the sign-in window.)
- Click on **Chart** and then on **204** for Maggie Gardner's chart. (*Remember:* You are not able to visit patients or administer medications during Period of Care 4. You are able to review patient records only.)
- Review the **History and Physical**.

1. How many losses related to pregnancy has Maggie Gardner experienced?

 • Click on the **Nursing Admission**.

2. What is the first evidence you find that Maggie Gardner's previous losses are affecting her current pregnancy and care? (*Hint*: Review the first five sections.)

→ • Click on the **Consultations** tab.

3. To what does Maggie Gardner attribute her inability to have a child?

4. List three therapeutic measures the chaplain can use to assist her through these feelings as part of her grieving process.

5. What did the chaplain accomplish during his time with Maggie Gardner?

Exercise 3

 Virtual Hospital Activity

 15 minutes

 Review the section on grief and loss in your textbook.

1. The grief response is closely linked to the _____ of the mother or father who has experienced the loss.

2. What are the four tasks of grief? (*Hint:* Consider Kübler-Ross theory.)

3. What are the three phases of grief?

4. List some physical symptoms that may manifest during the grieving process.

5. What response typically emerges during intense grief? Why?

6. List three other emotions that are experienced during the time period of intense grief.

7. During the phase of reorganization, what is the most common question? Explain.

- Sign in to work at Pacific View Regional Hospital on the Obstetrics Floor for Period of Care 4. (*Note:* If you are already in the virtual hospital from a previous exercise, click on **Leave the Floor** and then **Restart the Program** to get to the sign-in window.)
- Click on **Chart** and then on **204**. (*Remember:* You are not able to visit patients or administer medications during Period of Care 4. You are able to review patient records only.)
- Review the **History and Physical**.

8. You have now reviewed Maggie Gardner's History and Physical and compared her information with your textbook's discussion of what happens during the reorganization phase. What correlation do you see?

- Click on **Consultations**.
- Scroll down to review the Pastoral Care Spiritual Assessment.

9. Culture and religion play very large roles in how individuals handle a loss. How has Maggie Gardner handled her losses? (*Hint*: See the Spirituality/Faith Factors section of this consult.)

LESSON 13

Medication Administration

Patients: Dorothy Grant, Room 201
Stacey Crider, Room 202
Maggie Gardner, Room 204
Laura Wilson, Room 206

Objective:

• Correctly administer selected medications to obstetric patients, observing the six rights.

Exercise 1

 Virtual Hospital Activity

 30 minutes

Dorothy Grant was admitted at 30 weeks gestation for observation following blunt abdominal trauma (she was kicked in the abdomen). She is bleeding vaginally and may have sustained a placental abruption. Your assignment for this exercise is to give Rho(D) immune globulin to her.

• Sign in to work at Pacific View Regional Hospital on the Obstetrics Floor for Period of Care 2. (*Note*: If you are already in the virtual hospital from a previous exercise, click on **Leave the Floor** and then **Restart the Program** to get to the sign-in window.)
• From the Patient List, select Dorothy Grant (Room 201).

 Read about Rho(D) immune globulin on page 503 in your textbook.

1. Rho(D) immune globulin is a solution of _____ that contains _____.

   Rho(D) immune globulin is given to _____

   who has had a _____.

   Rho(D) immune globulin prevents sensitization by _____

   _____.

2. All of the following are reasons that Rho(D) immune globulin might be administered. Place an X next to the reason it has been ordered for Dorothy Grant.

_____ Within 72 hours of giving birth to an Rh-positive infant

_____ Prophylactically at 28 weeks gestation

_____ Following an incident or exposure risk that occurs after 28 weeks gestation

_____ During first trimester pregnancy following miscarriage or elective abortion or ectopic pregnancy

3. List the information about Dorothy Grant that must be determined before giving her Rho(D) immune globulin.

➡ • Click on **Go to Nurses' Station**.
   • Click on **Chart** and then on **201**.
   • Click on **Physician's Orders**.
   • Scroll to the orders for Wednesday 0730.

4. Write the physician's order for Rho(D) immune globulin.

5. According to your textbook, is this the correct dosage and route?

➡ • Click on **Laboratory Reports**
   • Locate the results for 0245 Wednesday.
   • Scroll down to find the type and screen results.

6. Dorothy Grant's blood type is _____.

7. What additional information do you need? Why? Is that information available?

- Click on **Return to Nurses' Station**.
- Click on **Medication Room**.
- Click on **Refrigerator**; then click on the refrigerator door to open it.
- Click on **Rho(D) Immune Globulin**.
- Click on **Put Medication on Tray**.
- Click on **Close Door** at the bottom of the screen.
- Click on **View Medication Room**.
- Click on **Preparation**.
- Click on **Prepare** and follow the Preparation Wizard prompts to complete preparation of Dorothy Grant's Rho(D) immune globulin dose. When the Preparation Wizard has finished asking questions, click **Finish**.
- Click on **Return to Medication Room**.
- Click on **201** to go to Dorothy Grant's room.
- Click on **Check Armband**.
- Click on **Patient Care**.
- Click on **Medication Administration**.

You are almost ready to give Dorothy Grant's injection. However, before you do . . .

8. Rho(D) immune globulin is often considered a blood product.
   a. True
   b. False

9. Suppose Dorothy Grant absolutely refuses to accept blood or blood products because of her religious beliefs. How would you handle the situation?

Now you're ready to administer the medication!

- Click on the down arrow next to **Select**; choose **Administer**.
- Follow the Administration Wizard prompts to administer Dorothy Grant's injection. Indicate **Yes** to document the injection in the MAR. When the Administration Wizard has finished asking questions, click **Finish**.
- Click on **Leave the Floor**.
- Click on **Look at Your Preceptor's Evaluation**.
- Click on **Medication Scorecard**. How did you do?
- Click on **Return to Evaluations**.
- Click on **Return to Menu**.

Exercise 2

  Virtual Hospital Activity

20 minutes

- Sign in to work at Pacific View Regional Hospital on the Obstetrics Floor for Period of Care 1. (*Note*: If you are already in the virtual hospital from a previous exercise, click on **Leave the Floor** and then **Restart the Program** to get to the sign-in window.)
- From the Patient List, select Maggie Gardner (Room 204).
- Click on **Go to Nurses' Station**.
- Click on the **Chart** and then on **204**.
- Click on the **Nursing Admission**.

1. Maggie Gardner verbalizes anxiety repeatedly throughout the Nursing Admission. What is her primary concern? Why? Provide documentation.

2. Maggie Gardner states that prior to this pregnancy she had a highly adaptive coping mechanism. How does she consider her ability to cope at this point? Why? (*Hint*: See the Coping and Stress Tolerance section in the Nursing Admission.)

 • Click on the **Physician's Orders**.

3. What medication has the physician ordered to help Maggie Gardner with her anxiety?

 • Click on **Return to Nurses' Station**.
- Click on the **Drug** icon in the lower-left corner of your screen.
- Use the Search box or the scroll bar to find the medication you identified in question 3.
- Review all of the information provided regarding this drug.

4. What is the drug's mechanism of action?

• Click on **Return to Nurses' Station**.
- Click on **204** to go to Maggie Gardner's room.
- Click on **Patient Care** and then **Nurse-Client Interactions**.
- Select and view the video titled **0745: Evaluation—Efficacy of Drugs**. (*Note:* Check the virtual clock to see whether enough time has elapsed. You can use the fast-forward feature to advance the time by 2-minute intervals if the video is not yet available. Then click on **Patient Care** and **Nurse-Client Interactions** to refresh the screen.)

5. According to the nurse, how long will it take for Maggie Gardner to see therapeutic effects? How does this correlate with what you learned in the Teaching Section of the Drug Guide?

Exercise 3

 Virtual Hospital Activity

 15 minutes

In this exercise, you will administer betamethasone to Stacey Crider, who was admitted to the hospital at 27 weeks gestation in preterm labor.

- Sign in to work at Pacific View Regional Hospital on the Obstetrics Floor for Period of Care 1. (*Note*: If you are already in the virtual hospital from a previous exercise, click on **Leave the Floor** and then **Restart the Program** to get to the sign-in window.)
- From the Patient List, select Stacey Crider (Room 202).

1. Before preparing Stacey Crider's betamethasone, what do you need to do first?

 • Click on **Go to Nurses' Station**.
- Click on **Chart** and then on **202**.
- Click on **Physician's Orders**.
- Scroll until you find the order for betamethasone.

2. After verifying the physician's order, what is your next step?

➡ • Click on **Return to Nurses' Station**.
 • Click on **Medication Room**.
 • Click on **Unit Dosage**.
 • Click on drawer **202**.
 • Click on **Betamethasone**.
 • Click on **Put Medication on Tray**.
 • Click on **Close Drawer** at the bottom of the screen.
 • Click on **View Medication Room**.
 • Click on **Preparation**.
 • Click on **Prepare** and follow the Preparation Wizard prompts to complete preparation of Stacey Crider's betamethasone dose. When the Preparation Wizard has finished asking questions, click **Finish**.
 • Click on **Return to Medication Room**.

3. Now that the medication is prepared, what is your next step?

➡ • Click on **202** to go to the patient's room.
 • Click on **Check Armband**.
 • Click on **Check Allergies**.
 • Click on **Patient Care**.
 • Click on **Medication Administration**.
 • Click on the down arrow next to **Select** and choose **Administer**.
 • Follow the Administration Wizard prompts to administer Stacey Crider's betamethasone dose.

4. What is the final step in the process?

➡ • If you haven't already, indicate **Yes** to document the injection in the MAR. When the Administration Wizard has finished asking questions, click **Finish**.
 • Click on **Leave the Floor**.
 • Click on **Look at Your Preceptor's Evaluation**.
 • Click on **Medication Scorecard**. How did you do?
 • Click on **Return to Evaluations**.
 • Click on **Return to Menu**.

Exercise 4

Virtual Hospital Activity

30 minutes

- Sign in to work at Pacific View Regional Hospital on the Obstetrics Floor for Period of Care 1. (*Note*: If you are already in the virtual hospital from a previous exercise, click on **Leave the Floor** and then **Restart the Program** to get to the sign-in window.)
- From the Patient List, select Laura Wilson (Room 206).
- Click on **Go to Nurses' Station**.
- Click on **MAR**.
- Click on the tab for Room **206**.

1. Laura Wilson's medications for Wednesday include several different types of drugs. In the list below, place an X next to the one that is used to treat her HIV-positive status.

   _____ Zidovudine 200 mg PO every 8 hours

   _____ Prenatal multivitamin 1 tablet PO daily

   _____ Lactated Ringer's 75 mL/hr IV continuous

- Click on **Return to Nurses' Station**.
- Click on the **Drug** icon in the lower-left corner of the screen.
- Using the Search box or the scroll bar, find the drug you identified in question 1.

2. What is the drug's mechanism of action?

3. What is the drug's therapeutic effect?

4. Does this medication cross the placenta? Is it distributed in breast milk?

5. What symptoms/side effects of this medication need to be reported to the physician?

6. How should this medication be taken?

7. Your final assignment is to give Laura Wilson the medication that is due at 0800. During these lessons, we have provided you with the detailed instructions on how to give medications. Now it is time for you to fly solo. Don't forget the six rights of medication administration . . . and have fun!! Document below how you did.

If you'd like to get more practice, there are other medications that can be given at the beginning of the first three periods of care. Below is a list of the patients, the medications, the routes of administration, and the administration times you can use. As you practice, be sure to select the correct patient when you sign in. That way, you can get a Medication Scorecard for evaluation after you prepare and administer a medication. (*Remember:* If you need help at any time, refer to pages 19-22 and pages 26-35 in the **Getting Started** section of this workbook.)

PERIOD OF CARE 1

Room 201, Dorothy Grant

0730/0800—Betamethasone 12 mg IM

Prenatal multivitamin PO

Room 202, Stacey Crider

0800—Prenatal multivitamin PO

Metronidazole 500 mg PO

Betamethasone 12 mg IM

Insulin lispro Sub-Q

Nifedipine 20 mg PO

Room 203, Kelly Brady

0730/0800—Prenatal multivitamin PO

Ferrous sulfate PO

Labetalol hydrochloride 400 mg PO

Nifedipine 10 mg PO

Room 204, Maggie Gardner

0800—Prenatal multivitamin PO

Buspirone hydrochloride 7.5 mg PO

Room 205, Gabriela Valenzuela

0800—Ampicillin 2 g IV

Betamethasone 12 mg IM

Prenatal multivitamin PO

Room 206, Laura Wilson

0800—Zidovudine 200 mg PO

Prenatal multivitamin PO

PERIOD OF CARE 2

Room 201, Dorothy Grant

1200—Rho(D) immune globulin IM

Room 202, Stacey Crider

1200—Insulin lispro Sub-Q

Room 203, Kelly Brady

1130—Betamethasone 12 mg IM

Room 204, Maggie Gardner

1115—Prednisone 40 mg PO

Aspirin 81 mg PO

PERIOD OF CARE 3

Room 204, Maggie Gardner

1500—Buspirone 7.5 mg PO

LESSON **14**

Care of the Infant with Respiratory Distress

 Reading Assignment: Communication, History, and Physical Assessment (Chapter 29): Lungs

Pediatric Variations of Nursing Interventions (Chapter 39): Procedures for Maintaining Respiratory Function; Inhalation Therapy; Administration of Medication—Oral Administration

Respiratory Dysfunction (Chapter 40): Respiratory Syncytial Virus (RSV) and Bronchiolitis

Gastrointestinal Dysfunction (Chapter 41): Dehydration

Pediatric Vital Signs and Parameters (Appendix C)

Patient: Carrie Richards, Room 303

Objectives:

- Recognize signs of acute respiratory distress in an infant.
- Describe interventions to treat respiratory distress in an infant.
- Describe the nursing care of an infant with RSV/bronchiolitis.

Exercise 1

Clinical Preparation: Writing Activity

15 minutes

1. What is RSV? Briefly describe the characteristic progression of this illness in children. Also identify any associated clinical manifestations.

2. How is this illness transmitted?

3. Describe the steps that can be taken to reduce or prevent the transmission of this illness.

4. List four priority nursing interventions for an infant with RSV.

5. What prophylactic medication is given to prevent RSV/bronchiolitis?

   a. How is this medication administered?

   b. When should this medication be administered?

   c. Given Carrie's history of birth and current illness, describe her status as a candidate to receive this prophylactic medication. Provide a rationale. (*Hint:* See History and Physical.)

Exercise 2

Virtual Hospital Activity

45 minutes

- Sign in to work at Pacific View Regional Hospital on the Pediatrics Floor for Period of Care 1. (*Note:* If you are already in the virtual hospital from a previous exercise, click on **Leave the Floor** and then **Restart the Program** to get to the sign-in window.)
- From the Patient List, select Carrie Richards (Room 303).
- Click on **Go to Nurses' Station**.
- Click on **Chart** and then on **303** for Carrie's chart.
- Click on **Emergency Department** and review this record.

1. What are Carrie's vital signs on admission to the ED at 1630? Which findings are out of normal range for a child her age?

2. Briefly describe the findings for Carrie recorded in the ED Systems Review and in the ED Nurse's Notes at 1800. Put an asterisk next to any findings that are abnormal for a child Carrie's age.

3. List the five cardinal clinical signs of respiratory distress (RD) in an infant.

→ • Still in the Emergency Department section of the chart, compare the findings in the ED Nurse's Notes at 1800 and 1900.

4. What clinical signs documented by the nurse indicate a change in Carrie's respiratory status at 1900?

5. What specific intervention is performed to improve Carrie's oxygenation status?

6. What medication is administered to Carrie to improve her respiratory status in the ED?

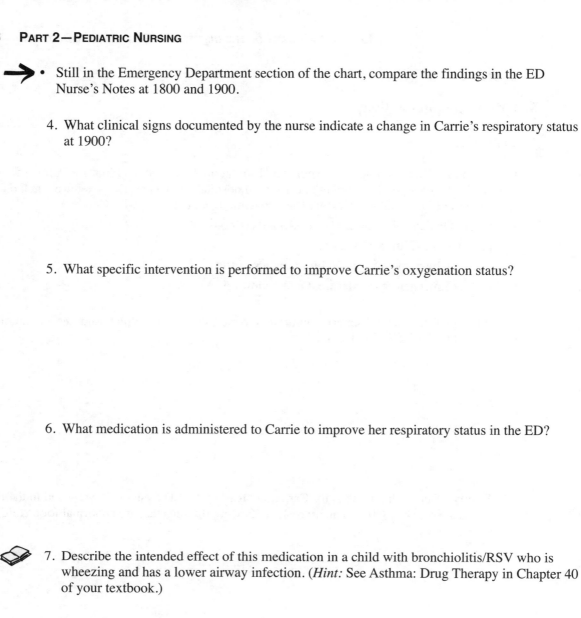 7. Describe the intended effect of this medication in a child with bronchiolitis/RSV who is wheezing and has a lower airway infection. (*Hint:* See Asthma: Drug Therapy in Chapter 40 of your textbook.)

8. Describe how this medication is administered in an infant Carrie's age. What is the rationale for this method of administration? (*Hint:* Refer to the Drug Guide.)

9. List two side effects of this medication for which the nurses should be vigilant.

10. Identify priority nursing assessments that need to be performed after the nebulizer treatment is given.

11. What is the primary medical diagnosis listed for Carrie?

12. List two nursing diagnoses for Carrie based on your review of her status in the ED.

13. In the 1800 ED Nurse's Notes, an important clue is given in relation to the severity of Carrie's status. What might lead you to conclude that her condition is poor? (*Hint:* Consider her age and developmental status.)

→ • Still in Carrie's chart, click on **Laboratory Reports**.

14. Below, fill in Carrie's laboratory values recorded in the ED at 1800 on Tuesday.

Chemistry	Arterial Blood Gas
Glucose	pH
Sodium (serum)	PaO_2
Potassium	$PaCO_2$
Chloride	Oxygen sat
CO_2 (serum)	
Creatinine	
BUN	
Calcium	

Urinalysis	Hematology
Color	WBC
Clarity	RBC
Glucose	Hgb
Bilirubin	Hct
Blood	Platelets
Spec gravity	Differential
pH	Segs
Protein	Bands
Ketones	Lymphocytes
WBC	Monocytes
	Eosinophils
	Basophils

 15. Which lab values in the table in question 14 are out of normal range for a child Carrie's age? (*Hint:* See Appendix D, Common Laboratory Tests, in your textbook.)

→ • Click on **Emergency Department**. Once again, review the ED Nurse's Notes for 1900 on Tuesday.

16. How is Carrie's respiratory status described? What interventions other than the nebulized medication administration and oxygen were performed to improve Carrie's respiratory status? State the rationale for the intervention performed.

 17. List the clinical signs, physical assessment findings, and any laboratory values that provide a basis for determining Carrie's hydration status on admission to the ED. (*Hint:* You may also refer to Dehydration in Chapter 41, as well as Parenteral Fluid Therapy in Chapter 39 of your textbook.)

 18. Based on Carrie's physical assessment findings, history, and current lab values, which type of dehydration is she manifesting? (*Hint:* Refer to Types of Dehydration in Chapter 41 of your textbook.)

    a. Isotonic
    b. Hypotonic
    c. Hypertonic

19. Describe the intervention(s) used to hydrate Carrie in the ED.

20. List two reasons Carrie is not a candidate for oral hydration in the ED.

21. Describe important assessment data that should be documented regarding the child's IV site.

→ • Still in Carrie's chart, click on and review the **Nursing Admission** and **History and Physical**.

22. List two modifiable health-related risk factors that place Carrie at high risk for the development of RSV.

23. List two socioeconomic factors that place Carrie at high risk for the development of RSV.

LESSON 15

Care of the Hospitalized Infant

Reading Assignment: Communication, History, and Physical Assessment (Chapter 29): Lungs

Pediatric Variations of Nursing Interventions (Chapter 39): Controlling Elevated Temperatures

Respiratory Dysfunction (Chapter 40): Respiratory Syncytial Virus (RSV) and Bronchiolitis

Patient: Carrie Richards, Room 303

Objectives:

- Perform a physical assessment of an infant with respiratory distress.
- Describe the nursing care of an infant with RSV/bronchiolitis.

Exercise 1

 Virtual Hospital Activity

 20 minutes

- Sign in to work at Pacific View Regional Hospital on the Pediatrics Floor for Period of Care 1. (*Note:* If you are already in the virtual hospital from a previous exercise, click on **Leave the Floor** and then **Restart the Program** to get to the sign-in window.)
- From the Patient List, select Carrie Richards (Room 303).
- Click on **Get Report**.
- Click on **Go to Nurses' Station**.
- Click on **Chart** and then on **303**.
- Click on and review the **Emergency Department** records.
- Click on and review the **History and Physical**.
- Click on and review the **Nursing Admission** and the **Physician's Orders** for Tuesday 1700 and 2300.

1. Briefly summarize Carrie's health history since birth.

 2. Is Carrie's immunization status current? If not, list the immunization(s) she should receive as soon as possible. (*Hint:* See Immunizations in Chapter 31 of your textbook.)

3. Based on Carrie's present respiratory illness, what immunization should she receive when she is 6 months old that may help protect her from further serious respiratory illnesses?

 • Before leaving the chart, record Carrie's physical assessment findings on admission in the middle column of the table in question 3. (*Hint:* You can find these in the Emergency Department record.)
• Click on **Return to Nurses' Station**.
• Click on **303** to go to Carrie's room.
• Click on **Patient Care** and then **Physical Assessment**.
• Perform a focused assessment by selecting the various body areas (yellow boxes) and system subcategories (green boxes) as needed to complete question 3.

4. Record your findings from the physical assessment in the far-right column below. Then compare these current findings with those obtained on admission to the ED.

Findings	Admission 1700 Tuesday	Current Findings
Respiratory effort		
Breath sounds		
Adventitious lung sounds		
Sensory/activity level		
Capillary refill		
Pulses		
Supplemental oxygen		

• Still in Carrie's room, click on **Patient Care** and then **Nurse-Client Interactions**.
• Select and view the video titled **0730: Patient Assessment**. (*Note:* Check the virtual clock to see whether enough time has elapsed. You can use the fast-forward feature to advance the time by 2-minute intervals if the video is not yet available. Then click on **Patient Care** and **Nurse-Client Interactions** to refresh the screen.)

5. How does the nurse assess Carrie's respiratory status in the video?

6. Carrie is 3½ months old. At this age, breathing is primarily:
   a. abdominal.
   b. diaphragmatic.

 • Click on **Take Vital Signs**.

7. Record Carrie's vital sign results below.

Temperature

Heart rate

Respiratory rate

Oxygen saturation

Blood pressure

8. Based on Carrie's current physical assessment findings and vital signs, what conclusion might be drawn about her respiratory status and general health at this time?

• Click on **EPR** and **Login**.
• Select **303** as the patient's room.
• Choose various categories as needed to record the vital signs and physical assessment findings you gathered in Carrie's room. Be sure to include respiratory findings and IV status.

Exercise 2

Virtual Hospital Activity

 45 minutes

- Sign in to work at Pacific View Regional Hospital on the Pediatrics Floor for Period of Care 3. (*Note:* If you are already in the virtual hospital from a previous exercise, click on **Leave the Floor** and then **Restart the Program** to get to the sign-in window.)
- From the Patient List, select Carrie Richards (Room 303).
- Click on **Go to Nurses' Station**.
- Click on **Chart** and then on **303**.
- Review the **Nurse's Notes**.
- Click on **Return to Nurses' Station**.
- Click on **EPR** and then **Login**.
- Select **303** as the patient and **Respiratory** as the category.

1. Summarize Carrie's respiratory status at 1300 on Wednesday based on the 1240 Nurse's Notes and 1215 respiratory assessment data in the EPR.

 • Still in the EPR, change the category to **Vital Signs**.

2. What is Carrie's body temperature at 1445?

• Click on **Exit EPR**.
• Click on **MAR** and then on tab **303**.

3. What medication does Carrie have ordered for fever or irritability?

Now let's go to the Medication Room and prepare to administer all of the 1500 medications ordered for Carrie.

- First, click on **Return to Nurses' Station**.
- Next, click on **Medication Room**.
- Click on **MAR** to determine what medications Carrie should receive for 1500. You may review the MAR at any time to verify the correct medication order. (*Hint:* Remember to look at the patient name on the MAR to make sure you have the correct record—you must click on the tab with Carrie's room number within the MAR.) Click on **Return to Medication Room** after reviewing the correct MAR.
- Click on **Unit Dosage** and then on drawer **303**.
- Select the medications you would like to administer. For each medication you select, click on **Put Medication on Tray**. When you are finished, click on **Close Drawer**.
- Click **View Medication Room**.
- Now click on **Automated System** and **Login**.
- Select the correct patient and drawer according to the medication you want to administer. (*Hint:* This automated system is for controlled substances only.) Then click **Open Drawer**.
- Select the medication you would like to administer, click on **Put Medication on Tray**, and then click **Close Drawer**.
- Click **View Medication Room**.
- Click on **Preparation** and select the medication to administer.
- Click **Prepare** and wait for the Preparation Wizard to appear. If the Wizard requests information, provide your answer(s) and then click **Next**.
- Choose the correct patient and then click **Finish**.
- Repeat the previous three steps until all medications that you want to administer are prepared.
- You can click on **Review Your Medications** and then click **Return to Medication Room** when ready. When back in the Medication Room, go directly to Carrie's room by clicking on **303** at the bottom of the screen.
- In Carrie's room, administer the medications, utilizing the rights of medication administration. After you have collected the appropriate assessment data and are ready for administration, click **Patient Care** and then **Medication Administration**. Verify that the correct patient and medication(s) appear in the left-hand window. Then click the down arrow next to Select. From the drop-down menu, select **Administer** and complete the Administration Wizard by providing any information requested. When the Wizard stops asking for information, click **Administer to Patient**. Specify **Yes** when asked whether this administration should be recorded in the MAR. Finally, click **Finish**. Complete these steps for each medication you wish to administer.

Now let's see how you did!

- Click on **Leave the Floor** at the bottom of your screen. From the Floor Menu, select **Look at Your Preceptor's Evaluation**. Then click on **Medication Scorecard**.
- Review the scorecard to see whether or not you correctly administered the appropriate medication(s). If not, why do you think you were incorrect? According to Table C in this scorecard, what resources should be used and what important assessments should be completed before administering the medication(s)? Did you utilize these resources and perform these assessments correctly?
- Print a copy of the Medication Scorecard for your instructor to evaluate.

4. How does the nurse evaluate pain or discomfort in an infant Carrie's age? (*Hint:* See Pain Assessment in Chapter 30 of your textbook.)

5. What is the most appropriate behavioral pain scale to assess Carrie's pain?

➡ • Still in Carrie's room, click on **Patient Care** and then **Nurse-Client Interactions**.
   • Select and view the video titled **1500: Teaching—Oral Medication**. (*Note:* Check the virtual clock to see whether enough time has elapsed. You can use the fast-forward feature to advance the time by 2-minute intervals if the video is not yet available. Then click on **Patient Care** and **Nurse-Client Interactions** to refresh the screen.)

6. How does the nurse teach Carrie's mother to administer the oral medication?

7. What statement(s) does Carrie's mother make about Carrie's eating habits in the last few days prior to admission?

8. What interrelated factors should the nurse consider when an infant has a compromising respiratory illness, such as RSV/bronchiolitis, and the infant's food intake is decreased?

9. What are the implications of these findings for an infant in relation to hydration status and present illness? (*Hint:* See Water Balance in Infants in Chapter 41 of your textbook.)

10. What concerns does Carrie's mother express about her daughter's nutritional status?

11. How does the nurse address the mother's concerns about Carrie's nutritional status?

 12. An infant's illness and hospitalization may represent a significant stressor for a single mother and her infant. What can the nursing staff do to minimize Brenda's anxiety about Carrie's hospitalization? (*Hint:* See Preventing and Minimizing Separation in Chapter 38 of your textbook.)

16

Nutritional Assessment and Discharge Planning

 Reading Assignment: The Infant and Family (Chapter 31): Special Health Problems; Failure to Thrive

Family-Centered Care of the Child During Illness and Hospitalization (Chapter 38): Nursing Care of the Family; Preparing for Discharge and Home Care

Patient: Carrie Richards, Room 303

Objectives:

- Assess the nutritional status of the infant with suspected failure to thrive.
- Describe the nursing care of the infant with failure to thrive, including family interventions for home care and management.

Exercise 1

Virtual Hospital Activity

20 minutes

- Sign in to work at Pacific View Regional Hospital on the Pediatrics Floor for Period of Care 1. (*Note:* If you are already in the virtual hospital from a previous exercise, click on **Leave the Floor** and then **Restart the Program** to get to the sign-in window.)
- From the Patient List, select Carrie Richards (Room 303).
- Click on **Get Report**.
- Click on **Go to Nurses' Station**.
- Click on **Chart** and then on **303**.
- Click on and review the **Emergency Department** records for Carrie.
- Click on and review the **History and Physical**.
- Click on and review the **Nursing Admission** and the **Physician's Notes**.

1. What are Carrie's weight and length on admission to the ED? (*Hint:* See Nursing Admission and History and Physical.)

2. What observations are made regarding the appearance of Carrie's body size in the ED?

3. What additional observations are made by the staff that address Carrie's overall nutritional status?

4. What is Carrie's secondary medical diagnosis in the ED?

5. What is the rationale for weighing Carrie again on Wednesday morning at 0755?

6. On the following page, review the CDC/WHO growth chart entitled "Birth to 36 months: Girls—Length-for-age and Weight-for-age percentiles." Plot Carrie's admission weight and length on the chart.

   Carrie Richards is _____ for weight-for-age and roughly at the

   _____ for length-for-age.

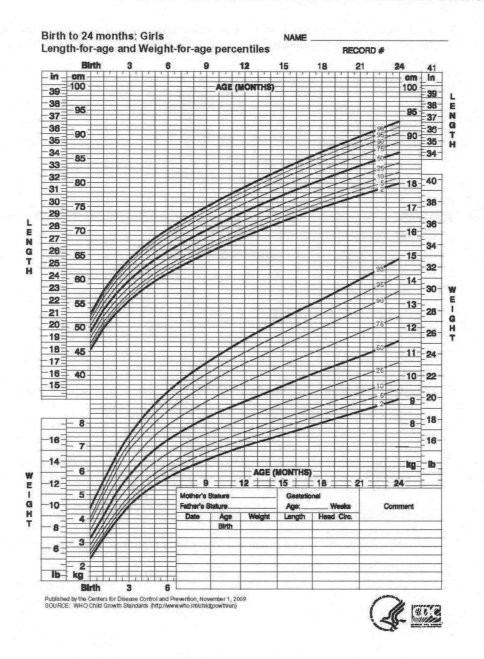

Birth to 24 months: Girls
Length-for-age and Weight-for-age percentiles

NAME _____

RECORD # _____

Published by the Centers for Disease Control and Prevention, November 1, 2009
SOURCE: WHO Child Growth Standards (http://www.who.int/childgrowth/en)

7. What is the significance of these findings for an infant her age?

→ • Once again, review Carrie's **History and Physical** and **Nursing Admission** in the chart.

8. In the dietary history there is significant information regarding Carrie's feedings. What does Carrie's mother say she has been feeding her daughter? (Include amounts and frequency as applicable.)

9. What is the significance of this information? (*Hint:* See Nutrition, The First 6 Months in Chapter 31 in your textbook.)

10. What is the rationale given for the addition of rice cereal to a nighttime bottle?

11. Is the practice of putting an infant to sleep with a nighttime bottle recommended? Why?

12. Briefly discuss the practice of feeding an infant Carrie's age solids before the age of 4 months. What are the possible health implications of feeding an infant solids at this early age?

• Click on **Return to Nurses' Station**.
- Click on **303** to go to Carrie's room.
- Click on **Patient Care** and then on **Nurse-Client Interactions**.
- Select and view the video titled **0800: Assessment—Fact Finding**. (*Note:* Check the virtual clock to see whether enough time has elapsed. You can use the fast-forward feature to advance the time by 2-minute intervals if the video is not yet available. Then click on **Patient Care** and **Nurse-Client Interactions** to refresh the screen.)

13. What does the nurse tell Carrie's mother she will do to assess Carrie's ability to tolerate feedings in relation to her condition?

14. What additional observations might the nurse make at the time of feeding?

15. How is the diagnosis of growth failure established? (*Hint:* See Failure to Thrive, Diagnostic Evaluation in Chapter 31 in your textbook.)

Exercise 2

 Virtual Hospital Activity

 25 minutes

- Sign in to work at Pacific View Regional Hospital on the Pediatrics Floor for Period of Care 2. (*Note:* If you are already in the virtual hospital from a previous exercise, click on **Leave the Floor** and then **Restart the Program** to get to the sign-in window.)
- From the Patient List, select Carrie Richards (Room 303).
- Click on **Go to Nurses' Station**.

- Click on **Chart** and then **303**.
- Click on **Consultations** and read the Dietary/Nutrition Consult.

1. What does the dietitian report regarding Carrie's nutritional status?

2. According to the consult findings, what additional information is discovered about how Carrie is fed that has a significant impact on the amount of calories she has been receiving?

3. How might the nurse assess the report that Carrie spits up frequently after feedings?

➤ • Click on **Chart** and then on **303**.
- Click on **Consultations**.
- In the Dietary Consult, review the dietitian's plan for Carrie to achieve catch-up growth in the next few weeks.
- Now click on **Nurse's Notes** and review the notes for Wednesday at 1240, 1425, and 1500.

4. Briefly summarize Carrie's feeding pattern since the acute phase of respiratory distress has resolved and her breathing has improved.

5. Write two measurable outcomes for weight gain and caloric (formula) intake for Carrie for the next few days. How will these outcomes be measured?

6. Some interventions have been addressed dealing with Carrie's growth failure. Identify additional nursing interventions that would be appropriate to implement in the hospital setting to help the mother care for Carrie.

Exercise 3

 Virtual Hospital Activity

 15 minutes

- Sign in to work at Pacific View Regional Hospital on the Pediatrics Floor for Period of Care 3. (*Note:* If you are already in the virtual hospital from a previous exercise, click on **Leave the Floor** and then **Restart the Program** to get to the sign-in window.)
- From the Patient List, select Carrie Richards (Room 303).
- Click on **Go to Nurses' Station**.
- Click on **Chart** and then on **303**.
- Click on **Consultations** and review the Social Service Consult at 1430 on Wednesday.
- While in the chart, also review the **Nursing Admission** and the **History and Physical**.

1. Describe Carrie's mother's family situation, marital status, sources of economic support, and any other factors that may influence her ability to care for herself and her daughter.

2. In addition to discharge teaching regarding nutrition, briefly discuss Carrie's risk status for sudden infant death syndrome and list at least five major points (modifiable risk factors) to be discussed with Brenda regarding the prevention of SIDS. (*Hint:* See Chapter 31, Sudden Infant Death Syndrome.)

3. Devise a plan for postdischarge follow-up for Carrie and her mother. Consider the mother's lack of transportation, the need for close medical follow-up to assess Carrie's progress over the next few weeks, and the limited family resources. Set up the plan for Carrie's discharge on Thursday morning, and evaluate the feasibility of the plan, assuming that her respiratory status continues to improve as it has since admission Tuesday evening.

LESSON 17

Emergent Care of the Hospitalized Child with Type 1 Diabetes Mellitus

 Reading Assignment: The School-Age Child and Family (Chapter 34)
Reaction to Illness and Hospitalization (Chapter 38):
Stressors of Hospitalization and Children's Reaction;
Later Childhood and Adolescence
Gastrointestinal Dysfunction (Chapter 41): Dehydration
Endocrine Dysfunction (Chapter 46): Disorders of Pancreatic
Hormone Secretion: Diabetes Mellitus

Patient: George Gonzalez, Room 301

Objectives:

- Recognize the clinical manifestations of diabetic ketoacidosis (DKA) in a child with type 1 diabetes mellitus.
- Describe the pathophysiology of diabetic ketoacidosis in a child with type 1 diabetes mellitus.
- Describe the nursing care of the child with DKA.
- Identify significant diagnostic laboratory tests in the management of type 1 diabetes mellitus.

Exercise 1

 Virtual Hospital Activity

 30 minutes

- Sign in to work at Pacific View Regional Hospital on the Pediatrics Floor for Period of Care 1. (*Note:* If you are already in the virtual hospital from a previous exercise, click on **Leave the Floor** and then **Restart the Program** to get to the sign-in window.)
- From the Patient List, select George Gonzalez (Room 301).
- Click on **Go to Nurses' Station**.
- Click on **Chart** and then on **301** for George Gonzalez's record.
- Click on **Emergency Department**.

1. What were George Gonzalez's primary and secondary medical diagnoses on admission to the ED?

2. List four clinical manifestations of DKA.

3. What is the significance of vomiting in a child who has DKA?

4. List altered neurologic signs the nurse should be alert for in a child with DKA. (*Hint:* See Table 46-3 in your textbook.)

• Click on **Laboratory Reports** and review the initial lab work drawn in the ED at 1730 on Tuesday.

5. What was George Gonzalez's blood glucose result on admission?

6. List the normal blood glucose values for a child George Gonzalez's age. (*Hint:* See Appendix D in your textbook.)

7. Complete the table below with George Gonzalez's lab values and normal parameters.

Lab Values	George's Values	Normal Values
Sodium (serum)		
Potassium (serum)		
BUN		
Creatinine		
CO_2 (serum)		
Urine ketones		
Urine glucose		
Urine specific gravity		
Arterial pH		
$PaCO_2$		
PaO_2		
WBC		
Hgb		
Hct		
Platelets		
RBC		

8. In addition to an elevated serum glucose, which of George's lab values support the diagnosis of DKA?

9. Briefly discuss the relationship between dehydration, DKA, and George's lab values that support this diagnosis.

10. Identify the initial intervention performed in the ED to rehydrate George Gonzalez.

11. What nursing observations are particularly important for a child with DKA who is receiving intravenous fluids? (*Hint:* See Nursing Care Management of DKA in Chapter 46 of your textbook.)

12. What is the significance of monitoring cardiac function in a child with DKA?

• Click on **Physician's Orders** and review the orders for George Gonzalez in the ED at 1730.

13. What medication is ordered?

To answer the following questions, refer to the Diabetes Mellitus section of Chapter 46 in your textbook.

14. What is the preferred method for administering insulin to a patient with DKA?

15. How was George Gonzalez's insulin administered in the ED at 1730?

16. What is the significance of admitting a child with DKA to an intensive care unit?

17. What are Kussmaul respirations?

18. What is the significance of Kussmaul respirations in ketoacidosis?

LESSON 18

Care of the Hospitalized Child with Type 1 Diabetes Mellitus

Reading Assignment: Endocrine Dysfunction (Chapter 46): Disorders of Pancreatic
Hormone Secretion: Diabetes Mellitus

Patient: George Gonzalez, Room 301

Objectives:

- Identify clinical manifestations of type 1 diabetes mellitus.
- Differentiate among the types of insulin used in the child with type 1 diabetes mellitus.
- Identify specific learning and emotional needs of the preadolescent with a chronic illness.

Exercise 1

  Virtual Hospital Activity

35 minutes

- Sign in to work at Pacific View Regional Hospital on the Pediatrics Floor for Period of
  Care 1. (*Note:* If you are already in the virtual hospital from a previous exercise, click on
  Leave the Floor and then **Restart the Program** to get to the sign-in window.)
- From the Patient List, select George Gonzalez (Room 301).
- Click on **Go to Nurses' Station**.
- Click on **Chart** and then on **301** for George Gonzalez's record.
- Review the **History and Physical** and **Nursing Admission** sections of the chart.

1. List the three "Ps" that are cardinal signs associated with type 1 diabetes mellitus. Briefly
   explain the significance of each term. Put an asterisk next to the signs that George Gonzalez
   demonstrated prior to his admission.

2. In the table below list the clinical manifestations of type 1 diabetes mellitus.

Clinical Manifestations

Nutrition/Diet

Neurologic/Mental

Metabolic/Endocrine

Genitourinary

Activity

Other

3. Diabetes mellitus (DM) may mimic other illnesses and may be overlooked. What are some of the accompanying signs and symptoms that may cause one to overlook DM?

4. What was George Gonzalez's $HgbA_{1C}$ (glycosylated hemoglobin) on admission to the ED?

5. The primary goals of DM treatment are to maintain glucose levels less than _____ mg/dL

and a glycosylated hemoglobin ($HgbA_{1C}$) less than _____ %.

6. What is the significance of the $HgbA_{1C}$ in a person with diabetes mellitus in relation to compliance and long-term complications?

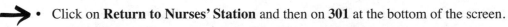

- Click on **Return to Nurses' Station** and then on **301** at the bottom of the screen.
- Click on **Patient Care** and then **Nurse-Client Interactions**.
- Select and view the video titled **0730: Supervision—Glucose Testing**. (*Note:* Check the virtual clock to see whether enough time has elapsed. You can use the fast-forward feature to advance the time by 2-minute intervals if the video is not yet available. Then click on **Patient Care** and **Nurse-Client Interactions** to refresh the screen.)

7. What does George Gonzalez say about checking his glucose at home?

8. What skill does the nurse ask George Gonzalez to perform during this interaction?

9. What is the significance of the nurse observing George Gonzalez check his glucose instead of her checking it for him?

10. What was George Gonzalez's fingerstick blood glucose at 0745 on Wednesday?

- Click on **Chart** and then on **301**.
- Click on **Physician's Orders** and review the orders written at 2200 on Tuesday.
- Click on **Return to Room 301**.
- Now click on **MAR** and review George Gonzalez's MAR for Wednesday morning.

11. What intervention should occur once George Gonzalez has checked his blood glucose level prebreakfast?

12. In addition to monitoring his glucose levels, what additional psychomotor skill should George Gonzalez be expected to perform in relation to diabetic management?

13. List the doses and types of insulin George Gonzalez is to administer before his breakfast.

14. What is the rationale for using both types of insulin throughout the day?

15. What step should be taken to prevent hypoglycemia when a rapid-acting insulin is administered?

Insulin is now available in a number of premixed forms that make administration easier. These forms include the insulin pump and insulin pen. The insulin pump and pen may not be available to all children because of cost and skill level. George Gonzalez may be a candidate for administering insulin with an insulin pen.

16. Briefly describe the advantages of an insulin pen for a person of George Gonzalez's age.

17. Match each type of insulin below with its corresponding characteristics.

_____ Humalog (lispro H)   a. Rapid-acting insulin
        NovoLog (aspart)
                                  b. Intermediate-acting insulin
_____ NPH or Lente
                                  c. Long-acting insulin
_____ Regular

_____ UltraLente

_____ Lantus (glargine)

→ • Click on **Return to Room 301**.
  • Click on **Patient Care** and then on **Nurse-Client Interactions**.
  • Select and view the video titled **0745: Self-Administering Insulin**. (*Note:* Check the virtual clock to see whether enough time has elapsed. You can use the fast-forward feature to advance the time by 2-minute intervals if the video is not yet available. Then click on **Patient Care** and **Nurse-Client Interactions** to refresh the screen.)

18. In the video, what specific task does the nurse ask George Gonzalez to perform?

19. In this video interaction, how does the nurse evaluate George Gonzalez's understanding of his diabetes?

20. Based on your observation of George Gonzalez's actions in this video and his responses to the nurse about his condition, what conclusions would you draw about George Gonzalez's knowledge regarding diabetes and his subsequent ability to perform glucose monitoring and insulin injection?

21. In the interactions with the nurse, George Gonzalez makes a statement about how he has managed his diabetes previously. What does he say about his daily monitoring of glucose and administration of insulin before going to school?

LESSON 19

Diabetes and Self-Care Management

ᴏᴏ **Reading Assignment:** The School-Age Child and Family (Chapter 34): Nutrition
Reaction to Illness and Hospitalization (Chapter 38):
  Stressors and Reactions of the Family of the Child Who Is
  Hospitalized
Endocrine Dysfunction (Chapter 46): Disorders of Pancreatic
  Hormone Secretion: Diabetes Mellitus

Patient: George Gonzalez, Room 301

Objectives:

- Describe the significance of glucose monitoring, diet, and exercise in the management of the child with type 1 diabetes mellitus.
- Discuss the impact of a chronic illness on the preadolescent child and family.
- Identify potential complications of type 1 diabetes in relation to poor glycemic control.
- Identify specific learning needs of the preadolescent with a chronic illness.

Exercise 1

 Virtual Hospital Activity

 30 minutes

- Sign in to work at Pacific View Regional Hospital on the Pediatrics Floor for Period of Care 2. (*Note:* If you are already in the virtual hospital from a previous exercise, click on **Leave the Floor** and then **Restart the Program** to get to the sign-in window.)
- From the Patient List, select George Gonzalez (Room 301).
- Click on **Go to Nurses' Station**.
- Click on **Chart** and then on **301** for George Gonzalez's record.
- Click on and review the **Nurse's Notes** and **Physician's Notes**.
- Click on **Return to Nurses' Station** and then on **301** at the bottom of the screen to go to George Gonzalez's room.
- Click on **Patient Care** and then on **Nurse-Client Interactions**.

- Click on the videos titled **1115: Teaching—Disease Process** and **1130: Teaching—Managing Symptoms**. (*Note:* Check the virtual clock to see whether enough time has elapsed. You can use the fast-forward feature to advance the time by 2-minute intervals if the video is not yet available. Then click on **Patient Care** and **Nurse-Client Interactions** to refresh the screen.)

1. What does George Gonzalez's mother say about his diabetes management?

2. What does George Gonzalez's mother tell the nurse about recognizing his need for insulin?

3. The nurse discusses with George Gonzalez's mother signs indicating he may need insulin. What are the signs of hyperglycemia in a child George's age?

4. During these two video sessions, what evaluation is the nurse making regarding George Gonzalez's knowledge of diabetes management?

5. What does George Gonzalez tell the nurse about the signs of hypoglycemia and what he should do if he feels that he is hypoglycemic?

Note: To answer the following two questions you may need to return to Period of Care 1 and review the **Nurse-Client Interactions** with George Gonzalez and his mother. If you need help changing periods of care, see the **Getting Started** section of the workbook.

6. Briefly summarize your impressions regarding the following issues.

   a. George Gonzalez's previous management of diabetes in relation to glucose monitoring and insulin administration:

   b. George Gonzalez's mother's knowledge about the importance of daily diabetes management:

7. Briefly summarize the main teaching points the nurse has covered up to this point with George Gonzalez and his mother regarding diabetes management.

8. What could the nurse emphasize with George Gonzalez and his mother about diabetes management to help control his blood glucose and prevent further hospitalizations?

Exercise 2

 Virtual Hospital Activity

 45 minutes

- Sign in to work at Pacific View Regional Hospital on the Pediatrics Floor for Period of Care 3. (*Note:* If you are already in the virtual hospital from a previous exercise, click on **Leave the Floor** and then **Restart the Program** to get to the sign-in window.)
- From the Patient List, select George Gonzalez (Room 301).
- Click on **Go to Nurses' Station**.
- Click on **Chart** and then on **301** for George Gonzalez's record.
- Review the **History and Physical** and the **Nursing Admission**.
- Next, click on **Consultations** and review the Psychiatric Consult.

1. According to the History and Physical, George Gonzalez has been hospitalized for problems with diabetes. What specific problems has he had with diabetes management in the last 3 months?

2. List two nursing diagnoses for George Gonzalez based on what you have learned from his chart and the Nurse-Client Interactions viewed in the previous exercise.

3. Briefly describe George Gonzalez's family situation (parents, siblings, primary care provider).

4. There are insights to George Gonzalez's previous diabetes management patterns found in the Nursing Admission, History and Physical, and Psychiatric Consult in the chart. List four factors that contribute to George Gonzalez's noncompliance with the diabetes regimen in the last 4 months.

5. What involvement is expected of George Gonzalez's family, given his age and developmental stage? (*Hint:* See the Diabetes Mellitus Family Support section in Chapter 46 of your textbook.)

 6. George Gonzalez has had diabetes for 4 years. Briefly describe the effect of a chronic illness such as diabetes on a preadolescent and his family. (*Hint:* To learn more about the impact of illness or disability on the preadolescent, see Impact of the Child's Chronic Illness in Chapter 36 of your textbook.)

 • Review the Nutrition Consult.
• Click on **Return to Nurses' Station**.
• Click on **301** at the bottom of the screen to go to George Gonzalez's room.
• Inside his room, click on **Patient Care** and then on **Nurse-Client Interactions**.
• Select and view the video titled **1500: Teaching—Diabetic Diet**. (*Note:* Check the virtual clock to see whether enough time has elapsed. You can use the fast-forward feature to advance the time by 2-minute intervals if the video is not yet available. Then click on **Patient Care** and **Nurse-Client Interactions** to refresh the screen.)

7. What is George Gonzalez's recommended dietary intake?

8. What does the nurse discuss with George Gonzalez in regard to his food intake?

9. What has been George Gonzalez's pattern of eating in the last several months?

10. Describe the relationship of food intake to insulin injections in a child with type 1 DM.

➡ • Now select and view the video titled **1535: Teaching—Effects of Exercise**. (*Note:* Check the virtual clock to see whether enough time has elapsed. You can use the fast-forward feature to advance the time by 2-minute intervals if the video is not yet available. Then click on **Patient Care** and **Nurse-Client Interactions** to refresh the screen.)

11. What activity does George Gonzalez say he really likes?

12. Why is exercise an important part of the management of type 1 diabetes?

13. Identify important items in the following areas that the nurse should discuss with George Gonzalez in relation to diabetes management and exercise.

    a. Glucose monitoring

    b. Carbohydrate intake

    c. When not to exercise

    d. Signs of activity intolerance

14. What specific intervention does George Gonzalez promise to get involved in following discharge that is aimed at helping him manage his diabetes effectively?

Understanding Head Injury

──

 Reading Assignment: Reaction to Illness and Hospitalization (Chapter 38):
                                  Intensive Care Unit
                             Cerebral Dysfunction (Chapter 45): Cerebral Trauma;
                                  Head Injury

Patient: Tommy Douglas, Room 302

Objectives:

- Evaluate the pathophysiology related to acute head trauma in children.
- Participate in the care of a comatose child.
- Review medications given to a child who has experienced a head injury.

Exercise 1

 Virtual Hospital Activity

20 minutes

- Sign in to work at Pacific View Regional Hospital on the Pediatrics Floor for Period of Care 1. (*Note:* If you are already in the virtual hospital from a previous exercise, click on **Leave the Floor** and then **Restart the Program** to get to the sign-in window.)
- From the Patient List, select Tommy Douglas (Room 302).
- Click on **Go to Nurses' Station**.
- Click on **Chart** and then on **302**.
- Click on and review the **Nursing Admission**.

1. What are the clinical symptoms of increased intracranial pressure (ICP) in a child Tommy Douglas' age and in his current condition?

2. What is the definition of increased ICP?

3. List three causes of increased ICP.

4. Why is the concern for increased ICP important when caring for a patient with a head injury?

5. Which of the following vital sign changes are associated with brainstem injury following acute head trauma? Select all that apply.

_____ Rapid or intermittent respirations

_____ Wide fluctuations in pulse

_____ Widening pulse pressure

_____ Extreme fluctuations in blood pressure

_____ Elevated temperature

6. One of Tommy Douglas' nursing diagnoses is Risk for injury related to physical immobility, depressed sensorium, and intracranial pathology. List four nursing interventions for this nursing diagnosis specific to maintaining a stable ICP.

7. What is the expected outcome related to the nursing diagnosis in question 6?

Exercise 2

Virtual Hospital Activity

25 minutes

- Sign in to work at Pacific View Regional Hospital on the Pediatrics Floor for Period of Care 1. (*Note:* If you are already in the virtual hospital from a previous exercise, click on **Leave the Floor** and then **Restart the Program** to get to the sign-in window.)
- From the Patient List, select Tommy Douglas (Room 302).
- Click on **Go to Nurses' Station**.
- Click on **Chart** and then on **302**.
- Select the **Emergency Department** tab and review the ED admission notes.
- While in the chart, also click on and review the **Nurse's Notes** and the **History and Physical.**

1. What caused Tommy Douglas' head injury?

• Now click on **Expired MARs** and review Tommy Douglas' expired MAR for Sunday at 2300.

- Next, click on **Physician's Orders** and review orders written in the ED.
- For additional help with the following questions, consult the Drug Guide by first clicking on **Return to Nurses' Station** and then clicking either on the **Drug** icon in the lower left corner of the screen or on the **Drug Guide** itself on the counter.

2. Based on your knowledge of head injury, why did Tommy Douglas receive mannitol?

3. Describe the sequence of events from Tommy Douglas' admission to the Emergency Department to his admission to your unit. (*Hint:* For help, check the Nurse's Notes, Physician's Notes, and Physician's Orders sections of the chart.)

4. List three interventions specific to the treatment of a child with a head injury that were performed before Tommy Douglas' arrival on your unit.

LESSON 21

Assessing the Head-Injured Patient

👓 **Reading Assignment:** Communication, History, and Physical Assessment (Chapter 29):
Neurologic Assessment
Cerebral Dysfunction (Chapter 45): Cerebral Dysfunction

Patient: Tommy Douglas, Room 302

Objectives:

- Perform a neurologic assessment on a child who has experienced a head injury.
- Participate in the care of a comatose child.

Exercise 1

Virtual Hospital Activity

35 minutes

- Sign in to work at Pacific View Regional Hospital on the Pediatrics Floor for Period of Care 1. (*Note:* If you are already in the virtual hospital from a previous exercise, click on **Leave the Floor** and then **Restart the Program** to get to the sign-in window.)
- From the Patient List, select Tommy Douglas (Room 302).
- Click on **Go to Nurses' Station**.
- Click on **Chart** and then on **302** to access Tommy's chart.
- Click on **Emergency Department** and review the admission notes.
- Click on and review the **Nurse's Notes** and the **Physician's Notes**.

1. What are the three major components of the Glasgow Coma Scale?

2. In the following table, briefly describe how each of these diagnostic tests is performed. Then provide a rationale for each test to explain its use in assessing the extent of Tommy Douglas' head injury. (*Hint:* See Table 45-1: Neurologic Diagnostic Procedures in the textbook and diagnostic tests found in Tommy Douglas' medical record.)

Diagnostic Test	How Test Is Performed	Rationale for Test
Brain CT without contrast		
Skull x-ray		
Cervical spine x-ray (radiograph)		
Brain perfusion test		

Now let's assess Tommy Douglas' neurologic status over time since his admission to the ED. To do this, access and find neurologic assessment data in the following resources, recording your findings in the table as instructed in questions 3 and 4.

 • In the patient's chart, click on **Emergency Department** and review this report for Sunday admission.
• Next, click on **Physician's Notes** and review the notes for Monday 0930 and Tuesday 1730.
• Click on **Return to Nurses' Station**.
• Select **EPR** and click on **Login**.
• Specify **302** as the room number and **Neurologic** as the category.
• Review the neurologic findings for 0715 Wednesday.

3. In the table below, record the findings from your chart review of Tommy Douglas' neurologic status on Sunday, Monday, Tuesday, and Wednesday.

Neurologic Exam	Sunday Admission	Monday 0930	Tuesday 1730	Wednesday 0715
GCS: Total Score				
Pupils Right: Size				
Pupils Right: Reaction				
Pupils Left: Size				
Pupils Left: Reaction				
Cranial Nerves I-XII				
Orientation				
Perception and Cognition				
Mental Status				
Sensory				

- Click on **Exit EPR**.
- From the Nurses' Station click on **Leave the Floor**.
- At the Floor Menu, select **Restart the Program**.
- Sign in to work on the Pediatrics Floor for Period of Care 2.
- Again, select Tommy Douglas (Room 302) as your patient and click on **Go to Nurses' Station**.
- Now click on **EPR** and then on **Login**.
- Choose **302** as the patient's room and **Neurologic** as the category. Review the results of the neurologic assessment recorded on Wednesday at 0800.

4.

NEUROLOGIC ASSESSMENT

GLASGOW COMA SCALE					
Pupils	Right	Size			++ = Brisk
		Reaction			+ = Sluggish
	Left	Size			− = No reaction
		Reaction			C = Eye closed by swelling
Eyes open	Spontaneously	4			
	To speech	3			
	To pain	2			
	None	1			
Best motor response	Obeys commands	6			Usually record best arm or age-appropriate response
	Localizes pain	5			
	Flexion withdrawal	4			
	Flexion abnormal	3			
	Extension	2			
	None	1			

Pupil scale (mm): dots labeled 1 through 8

Best response to auditory and/or visual stimulus	>2 years		<2 years	
	Orientation	5	5 Smiles, listens, follows	
	Confused	4	4 Cries, consolable	
	Inappropriate words	3	3 Inappropriate persistent cry	
	Incomprehensible words	2	2 Agitated, restless	
	None	1	1 No response	
	Endotracheal tube or trach	T		

COMA SCALE TOTAL	

HAND GRIP:
Equal
Unequal
R____ L____
Weakness

LOC:
Alert/oriented x4
Sleepy
Irritable
Comatose
Disoriented
Combative
Lethargic
Awake
Sleeping
Drowsy
Agitated

MUSCLE TONE:
Normal
Arching
Spastic
Flaccid
Weak
Decorticate
Decerebrate
Other _____

EYE MOVEMENT:
Normal
Nystagmus
Strabismus
Other _____

FONTANEL/WINDOW:
Soft
Flat
Sunken
Tense
Bulging
Closed
Other _____

MOOD/AFFECT:
Happy
Content
Quiet
Withdrawn
Sad
Flat
Hostile

Complete the Glasgow Coma Scale readings below, using the findings from Tommy Douglas' neurologic examination at 0800 Wednesday morning.

Pupils right: size: _____

Pupils right: reaction: _____

Pupils left: size: _____

Pupils left: reaction: _____

Eyes open: _____

Best motor response: _____

Best response to auditory and or visual stimulus: _____

Endotracheal tube or trach: _____

Coma Scale total: _____

Hand grip: _____

LOC: _____

Muscle tone: _____

Eye movement: _____

Fontanel/window: _____

Mood/affect: _____

5. How did Tommy Douglas' neurologic assessment results change from early in his admission to the PICU (Monday) to his admission to the telemetry unit (Wednesday)? Document your findings below. (*Hint:* Go to the chart and review the Nurse's Notes and Physician's Notes.)

Monday

Wednesday

6. List the following activities in order of priority beginning with what you would assess first when examining a critically ill patient such as Tommy Douglas.

_____   Check intravenous fluids and lines

_____   Perform a physical assessment

_____   Check ventilator settings

_____   Obtain vital signs

LESSON 22

Acute Care Phase

Reading Assignment: Chronic Illness, Disability, and End-of-Life Care (Chapter 36): Perspectives on the Care of Children at the End of Life; Grief and Mourning
Reaction to Illness and Hospitalization (Chapter 38): Intensive Care Unit
Cerebral Dysfunction (Chapter 45): Cerebral Trauma

Patient: Tommy Douglas, Room 302

Objectives:

- Interpret physical assessment findings related to a child whose condition is unstable.
- Evaluate lab data of the child with a head injury.
- Observe interactions between health care providers and parents experiencing the loss of a child.
- Describe the diagnostic evaluation necessary to confirm brain death in a child.

Exercise 1

Virtual Hospital Activity

25 minutes

- Sign in to work at Pacific View Regional Hospital on the Pediatrics Floor for Period of Care 3. (*Note:* If you are already in the virtual hospital from a previous exercise, click on **Leave the Floor** and then **Restart the Program** to get to the sign-in window.)
- From the Patient List, select Tommy Douglas (Room 302).
- Click on **Go to Nurses' Station**.
- Click on **302** at the bottom of the screen to go to Tommy Douglas' room; then click on **Take Vital Signs**.
- Click on **EPR** and then **Login**.
- Select **302** from the Patient drop-down box as the patient's room and **Vital Signs** from the Category drop-down box as the category.
- Document Tommy Douglas' 1500 vital signs results in the EPR. (*Hint:* If you need help entering data in the EPR, see pages 15-16 in the **Getting Started** section of this workbook.)
- When you have finished entering these data, click on **Exit EPR**.

199

- Now click on **Chart** and then on **302**.
- Click on **Physician's Orders**.

1. Why were new orders written at this time?

 • Review Tommy Douglas' chart as needed to answer question 2.

2. In the left column below, list the tests used to establish brain death. In the right column, summarize the results of each of these tests for Tommy Douglas.

Diagnostic Test	Findings

 • Click on **Return to Room 302**.
- Click on **Patient Care**.
- Click on **Head & Neck**.
- Click on **Neurologic** in the green boxes and complete a neurologic assessment on Tommy Douglas.
- Now click on **EPR** and then on **Login**.
- Select **302** from the Patient drop-down box for Tommy Douglas' room and **Neurologic** from the Category drop-down box as the category.
- Scroll to locate the findings for Wednesday at 1400 and review.

3. Based on your review of the EPR and the in-room neurologic assessment, record Tommy Douglas' neurologic findings for Wednesday at 1400 in the table below and on the next page.

Neurologic Assessment	Findings—Wednesday 1400
Glasgow Coma Scale: Eyes	
Glasgow Coma Scale: Verbal	
Glasgow Coma Scale: Motor	
Glasgow Coma Total Score	

Neurologic Assessment	Findings—Wednesday 1400
Pupils Right: Size	
Pupils Right: Reaction	
Pupils Left: Size	
Pupils Left: Reaction	
Cranial Nerves I-XII	
Orientation	
Speech	
Cognitive and Perceptual	
Mental Status	
Sensation	

- Click on **Exit EPR**.
- Once again, observe Tommy Douglas' vital signs by clicking on **Take Vital Signs**.

4. Record Tommy's current vital signs below.

Vital Sign	Findings
Temperature (F)	
Systolic pressure	
Diastolic pressure	
BP mode of measurement	
Heart rate	
Respiratory rate	
SpO$_2$ (%)	

5. What do you observe to be continuing problem(s) for Tommy Douglas while waiting for organ procurement?

• Click on **Patient Care** and then on **Nurse-Client Interactions**.

- Select and view the video titled **1500: Nurse-Family Communication**. (*Note:* Check the virtual clock to see whether enough time has elapsed. You can use the fast-forward feature to advance the time by 2-minute intervals if the video is not yet available. Then click on **Patient Care** and **Nurse-Client Interactions** to refresh the screen.)

6. What was reinforced by the nurse during this conversation?

7. Why was it important for the nurse in the video interaction to discuss ways for the family to remember Tommy Douglas?

 • Now click on and view the video titled **1515: The Grieving Family**. (*Note:* Check the virtual clock to see whether enough time has elapsed. You can use the fast-forward feature to advance the time by 2-minute intervals if the video is not yet available. Then click on **Patient Care** and **Nurse-Client Interactions** to refresh the screen.)

8. Describe the role of a child life specialist and explain why this individual is an appropriate choice to meet with Tommy Douglas' siblings.

LESSON 23

Emergent Nursing Care of the Child with Meningitis

Reading Assignment: Communication, History, and Physical Assessment (Chapter 29): Neurologic Assessment

Cerebral Dysfunction (Chapter 45): Cerebral Dysfunction; Increased Intracranial Pressure (ICP); Neurologic Examination; Intracranial Infections; Bacterial Meningitis; Nonbacterial (Aseptic) Meningitis

Patient: Stephanie Brown, Room 304

Objectives:

- Analyze laboratory findings associated with childhood meningitis.
- Differentiate between bacterial and aseptic meningitis.
- Describe the components of a neurologic assessment for a child who is diagnosed with meningitis.
- Describe the pathophysiology of meningitis.

203

Exercise 1

 Clinical Preparation: Writing Activity

 10 minutes

1. Match the following terms with the corresponding characteristics.

_____ Meningitis	a. Viral inflammation of the meninges
_____ Mode of meningitis transmission	b. Majority of cases occur in children younger than 2 months of age
_____ Meningococcal meningitis	c. Vascular dissemination of mucosal organisms frequently from the nasopharyngeal site
_____ Bacterial meningitis	d. Pyogenic inflammation of the meninges
_____ Incidence of bacterial meningitis	e. Inflammation of the membranes covering the brain and spinal cord
_____ Aseptic meningitis	f. Occurs primarily in school-age children and adolescents

2. What are common clinical manifestations of meningitis in children and adolescents?

Exercise 2

 Virtual Hospital Activity

 45 minutes

- Sign in to work at Pacific View Regional Hospital on the Pediatrics Floor for Period of Care 1. (*Note:* If you are already in the virtual hospital from a previous exercise, click on **Leave the Floor** and then **Restart the Program** to get to the sign-in window.)
- From the Patient List, select Stephanie Brown (Room 304).
- Click on **Go to Nurses' Station**.
- Click on **304** at the bottom of the screen to go to Stephanie's room.
- Click on **Patient Care**.
- Click on **Head & Neck**.
- Click on **Neurologic** in the green boxes and view the assessment.

1. State the physiologic basis for Stephanie Brown's headache. (*Hint:* See section on Increased Intracranial Pressure in Chapter 45 of the textbook.)

- Click on **Chart** and then on **304**.
- Click on **Emergency Department** and review.
- Then, click on and read the **Nurse's Notes** and **Physician's Notes**.

2. List the clinical manifestations of meningitis exhibited by Stephanie Brown in the ED.

- Click on and read the **History and Physical** section of Stephanie Brown's chart.

3. Describe the Glasgow Coma Scale and list the three-part assessment of the coma scale.

- Click on **Laboratory Reports**. Review the findings recorded in the ED on Monday at 0100.

4. Below, list the abnormal findings you noted for Stephanie Brown in the Laboratory Reports. For each abnormal finding, give the normal range of results. Finally, what does each finding indicate? (*Hint:* Common laboratory tests are in Appendix B of the textbook).

Lab Test	Results	Normal Range	Indications

- Now click on **Diagnostic Reports** and review the summary of Stephanie Brown's lumbar puncture.

5. Below, list each of the cerebral spinal fluid (CSF) results from Stephanie Brown's lumbar puncture on Monday. For each finding, give the normal range of results and identify what each finding indicates. (*Hint:* Common laboratory tests are in Appendix B of the textbook.)

CSF (Lumbar)	Results	Normal Range	Indications

- Click on **Physician's Orders** and review.

6. What medication is ordered for Stephanie Brown for a high temperature?

7. What is the rationale for administering this medication by rectum (PR) in the ED at 0100 on Monday?

8. What is the rationale for having the head of Stephanie Brown's bed elevated 45 degrees?

9. Describe the standard isolation technique for a child with meningitis in an acute care center. (*Note:* You may describe the standard practice in an institution where you work as a staff member or student.)

 • Click on **Return to Nurses' Station**.
   • Click on **MAR**.
   • Click on tab **304** and review Stephanie Brown's records.

10. An intravenous infusion is started immediately in a child with suspected meningitis to administer IV fluids and:
   a. antiepileptic drugs.
   b. steroid drugs.
   c. blood products.
   d. antimicrobial drugs.

11. Provide a rationale for your answer in question 10.

Now let's go to the Medication Room and prepare to administer all of the 0730 and 0800 medications ordered for Stephanie Brown.

- First, click on **Return to Nurses' Station**.
- Next, click on **Medication Room** at the bottom of the screen.
- Click on **MAR** to determine what medications Stephanie Brown should receive for 0730 and 0800. You may review the MAR at any time to verify the correct medication order. (*Hint:* Remember to look at the patient name on the MAR to make sure you have the correct record—you must click on the tab with Stephanie Brown's room number within the MAR.) Click on **Return to Medication Room** after reviewing the correct MAR.
- Click on **Unit Dosage** and then on drawer **304**.
- Select the medications you would like to administer. For each medication you select, click on **Put Medication on Tray**. When you are finished, click on **Close Drawer** at the bottom of the screen.
- Click **View Medication Room**.
- Now click on **Automated System** and **Login**.
- Select the correct patient and drawer according to the medication you want to administer. (*Hint:* This automated system is for controlled substances only.) Then click **Open Drawer**.
- Select the medication you would like to administer, click on **Put Medication on Tray**, and then click **Close Drawer**.
- Click **View Medication Room**.
- Click on **Preparation** and select the medication to administer.
- Click **Prepare** and wait for the Preparation Wizard to appear. If the Wizard requests information, provide your answer(s) and then click **Next**.
- Choose the correct patient and then click **Finish**.
- Repeat the previous three steps until all medications that you want to administer are prepared.
- You can click on **Review Your Medications** and then click through the various tabs to review the ordered and prepared medications for Stephanie Brown. When you are ready, click **Return to Medication Room**. When back in the Medication Room, go directly to Stephanie Brown's room by clicking on **304** at the bottom of the screen.
- In Stephanie Brown's room, administer the medications, utilizing the rights of medication administration. After you have collected the appropriate assessment data and are ready for administration, click **Patient Care** and then **Medication Administration**. Verify that the correct patient and medication(s) appear in the left-hand window. Then click the down arrow next to Select. From the drop-down menu, select **Administer** and complete the Administration Wizard by providing any information requested. When the Wizard stops asking for information, click **Administer to Patient**. Specify **Yes** when asked whether this administration should be recorded in the MAR. Finally, click **Finish**. Complete these steps for each medication you wish to administer.

12. In the mock MAR form below, document the medications you administered.

Medication/Dose	2300-0700	0700-1500	1500-2300

13. Stephanie Brown is receiving maintenance IV fluids with strict fluid intake and output to prevent what severe complication?

 • To answer questions 14 through 16, you will need to consult the Drug Guide.
   • To access the Drug Guide, click on the **Drug** icon in the lower left corner of your screen. When the Drug Guide opens, use the Search box or scroll through the list of drugs at the top of the screen; select **vancomycin**.

14. Provide the rationale for the intravenous administration of this drug (versus oral administration).

15. Briefly describe the procedure for administering vancomycin intravenously to a child Stephanie Brown's age. Include the correct dilution, if required.

16. List three serious side effects for which the nurse should be vigilant during and after the administration of this medication.

Now let's see how you did administering Stephanie Brown's medications.

- Click on **Leave the Floor** at the bottom of your screen. From the Floor Menu, select **Look at Your Preceptor's Evaluation**. Then click on **Medication Scorecard**.
- Review the scorecard to see whether or not you correctly administered the appropriate medication(s). If not, why do you think you were incorrect? According to Table C in this scorecard, what resources should be used and what important assessments should be completed before administering the medication(s)? Did you utilize these resources and perform these assessments correctly?
- Print a copy of the Medication Scorecard for your instructor to evaluate.
- Click on **Return to Evaluations**.
- Click on **Return to Menu**.

LESSON 24

Nursing Care of the Hospitalized Child

 Reading Assignment: Pain Assessment and Management in Children (Chapter 30): Pain Assessment

Gastrointestinal Dysfunction (Chapter 41): Constipation

Cerebral Dysfunction (Chapter 45): Bacterial Meningitis

Patient: Stephanie Brown, Room 304

Objectives:

- Describe the nursing care of the child with meningitis and constipation.
- Identify the rationale for auditory testing in the child with meningitis.

Exercise 1

 Virtual Hospital Activity

45 minutes

- Sign in to work at Pacific View Regional Hospital on the Pediatrics Floor for Period of Care 2. (*Note:* If you are already in the virtual hospital from a previous exercise, click on **Leave the Floor** and then **Restart the Program** to get to the sign-in window.)
- From the Patient List, select Stephanie Brown (Room 304).
- Click on **Go to Nurses' Station**.
- Click on **Chart** and then on **304**.
- Click on **Emergency Department** and review this report.
- Click on and review the **Physician's Orders** and **Physician's Notes** for Wednesday at 0900.
- Click on **Return to Nurses' Station**.
- Click on **304** at the bottom of the screen to go to Stephanie Brown's room.
- Click **Patient Care** and then **Nurse-Client Interactions**.
- Select and view the video titled **1120: Preventing Spread of Disease**. (*Note:* Check the virtual clock to see whether enough time has elapsed. You can use the fast-forward feature to advance the time by 2-minute intervals if the video is not yet available. Then click on **Patient Care** and **Nurse-Client Interactions** to refresh the screen.)

1. What might explain why the physician decreased Stephanie Brown's IV rate to 10 mL/hr?

2. How did Stephanie Brown's nurse explain the basis for the respiratory isolation?

3. Based on your earlier review of the Physician's Notes, what was the physician's most likely rationale for discontinuing the respiratory isolation and vancomycin for Stephanie Brown?

→ • Still in Stephanie Brown's room, click on **Clinical Alerts** and review.

4. What does the Clinical Alert say regarding Stephanie Brown's abdominal assessment?

5. When did Stephanie Brown have her last bowel movement?

- Click on **Chart** and then **304**.
- Review the **Physician's Notes** to answer question 6.

6. Compare the Monday and Wednesday notes in regard to the Kernig sign, Brudzinski sign, and nuchal rigidity results for Stephanie Brown. Record any changes below. (*Hint:* See the Clinical Manifestation section in Chapter 45 of your textbook.)

- Click on **Return to Room 304**.
- Click on **MAR** and then on tab **304** to review Stephanie Brown's medication orders.

7. Are there further indications for performing an audiogram (hearing test) on this patient (besides the diagnosis of meningitis)?

- Click on **Return to Room 304**.
- Click on **Chart** and then on **304**.
- Click on **Physician's Orders** and review the orders for 1100 on Wednesday.

8. What medication is ordered for Stephanie Brown at this time?

- Click on **Return to Room 304**.
- Click on the **Drug** icon in the lower left corner of your screen.

9. Complete the following table for the drug you identified in question 8. Relate your answers specifically to Stephanie Brown's need for the medication.

Name of Medication	Classification	Action	Dosage	Frequency	Route

- Click on **Return to Room 304**.
- Click on **Medication Room** at the bottom of the screen.
- Click on **Unit Dosage** and then on **Drawer 304**.
- Select the medication that you would like to administer and click **Put Medication on Tray**. Click **Close Drawer** at the bottom of the screen and then click **View Medication Room**.
- Click on **Preparation** and then click **Prepare** next to the medication you identified in question 8.
- When you have finished the steps of the Preparation Wizard, click on **Return to Medication Room** and then on **304** at the bottom of the screen to go to Stephanie Brown's room.
- Administer the medication, utilizing the rights of medication administration. After you have collected the appropriate assessment data and are ready for administration, click **Patient Care** and then **Medication Administration**. Verify that the correct patient and medication(s) appear in the left-hand window. Then click the down arrow next to Select. From the drop-down menu, select **Administer** and complete the Administration Wizard by providing any information requested. When the Wizard stops asking for information, click **Administer to Patient**. Specify **Yes** when asked whether this administration should be recorded in the MAR. Finally, click **Finish**.

10. On the mock MAR below, document the medication you just administered to Stephanie Brown. Indicate the time you gave it in the correct column.

Medication/Dose	2300-0700	0700-1500	1500-2300

Now let's see how you did!

- Click on **Leave the Floor** at the bottom of your screen. From the Floor Menu, select **Look at Your Preceptor's Evaluation**. Then click on **Medication Scorecard**.
- Review the scorecard to see whether or not you correctly administered the appropriate medication. If not, why do you think you were incorrect? According to Table C in this scorecard, what resources should be used and what important assessments should be completed before administering the medication(s)? Did you utilize these resources and perform these assessments correctly?
- Print a copy of the Medication Scorecard for your instructor to evaluate.
- Click **Return to Evaluations**.
- Click **Return to Menu**.

In Chapter 30 of your textbook, review Table 30-3 and the sections titled Behavioral Measures and Physiologic Measures.

- Click **Return to Evaluations** and then **Return to Menu**.
- Click **Restart the Program** and sign in to work on the Pediatrics Floor for Period of Care 2.
- From the Patient List, select Stephanie Brown (Room 304).
- Click on **Go to Nurses' Station**.
- Click on **EPR** and then on **Login**.
- Select **304** from the Patient drop-down menu as the patient's room and **Vital Signs** from the Category drop-down menu as the category.

11. Compare Stephanie Brown's blood pressure and pain scale rating on Wednesday 0700 with her BP and pain rating on Wednesday at 1100.

12. Using the FACES pain rating scale below, place an X on the face that matches Stephanie Brown's description of her headache recorded on Wednesday at 1100.

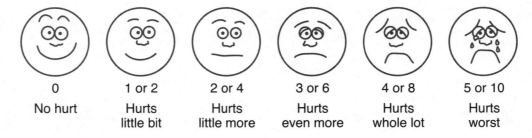

 • Click on **Exit EPR**.
   • Click on **Chart** and then on **304**.
   • Once again, review the **Physician's Orders** for Stephanie Brown.

13. What is ordered that can be administered to alleviate her headache?

 • Click on **Return to Nurses' Station**.
   • Now click on the **Drug** icon in the lower left corner of your screen.

14. Using the Drug Guide as your reference, complete the following table for the medication you identified in question 13.

Name of Medication	Classification	Action	Dose	Frequency	Route

 • Click on **Chart** and then on **304**.
   • Review the **Nurse's Notes** for Tuesday at 2300 and Wednesday at 0600.

15. Based on your assessment of Stephanie Brown at this time, what route would be appropriate for administering the medication you identified in question 13? State your rationale for choosing this route.

Nursing Care of the Hospitalized Child with Cerebral Palsy

Reading Assignment: Pain Assessment and Management in Children (Chapter 30): Transmucosal and Transdermal Analgesia

Reaction to Illness and Hospitalization (Chapter 38): Stressors of Hospitalization and Children's Reactions

Neuromuscular or Muscular Dysfunction (Chapter 49): Cerebral Palsy; Therapeutic Management

Patient: Stephanie Brown, Room 304

Objectives:

• Discuss the special needs of a child with cerebral palsy.
• Describe the issues involved in discharge planning and home care of the child with cerebral palsy.
• Identify measures to decrease anxiety in a child and family with meningitis.

Exercise 1

Virtual Hospital Activity

45 minutes

• Sign in to work at Pacific View Regional Hospital on the Pediatrics Floor for Period of Care 3. (*Note:* If you are already in the virtual hospital from a previous exercise, click on **Leave the Floor** and then **Restart the Program** to get to the sign-in window.)
• From the Patient List, select Stephanie Brown (Room 304).
• Click on **Go to Nurses' Station**.
• Click on **304** at the bottom of the screen to go to the patient's room.
• Click on **Patient Care** and then **Nurse-Client Interactions**.
• Select and view the video titled **1500: Assessment—IV Site**. (*Note:* Check the virtual clock to see whether enough time has elapsed. You can use the fast-forward feature to advance the time by 2-minute intervals if the video is not yet available. Then click on **Patient Care** and **Nurse-Client Interactions** to refresh the screen.)

1. How did the nurse describe the IV site in the video? What are the implications of her findings?

➤ • Now select and view the video titled **1510: Nurse-Patient Communication**. (*Note:* Check the virtual clock to see whether enough time has elapsed. You can use the fast-forward feature to advance the time by 2-minute intervals if the video is not yet available. Then click on **Patient Care** and **Nurse-Client Interactions** to refresh the screen.)

2. Describe the purpose of applying EMLA cream prior to restarting the IV as stated by the nurse in the video.

Let's take a virtual leap in time to see whether the EMLA cream was applied.

➤ • First, click on **Leave the Floor** and then on **Restart the Program**.
• Sign in to work on the Pediatrics Floor for Period of Care 4.
• Click on **MAR** and then on tab **304**. (*Remember:* You are not able to visit patients or administer medications during Period of Care 4. You are able to review patient records only.)
• Review Stephanie Brown's MAR for Wednesday at 1900.

3. At what time was the EMLA cream administered? Why should the nurse wait 60 minutes after EMLA is applied to the skin before the IV is restarted?

4. List two alternative (to EMLA) topical analgesics that would be appropriate to use on Stephanie Brown.

Now, let's return to Period of Care 3 to continue your care for Stephanie Brown.

- Click **Return to Nurses' Station** and once again, **Leave the Floor** and **Restart the Program**.
- Sign in to work on the Pediatrics Floor for Period of Care 3. Select Stephanie Brown (Room 304) from the Patient List.
- Click on **Go to Nurses' Station**.
- Click on **Chart** and then on **304**.
- Click on **History and Physical** and review.
- Click on **Nursing Admission** and review.

5. List the predisposing maternal and perinatal factors in Stephanie Brown's history that may have contributed to the development of cerebral palsy (CP).

6. What are the primary clinical problems noted in children with cerebral palsy that interfere with their ability to perform activities of daily living? (*Hint:* See Chapter 49, Cerebral Palsy.)

7. Using the Nursing Admission and History and Physical, describe two findings from the chart that relate to Stephanie's ability to perform ADLs.

8. Briefly describe the indication(s) for administering baclofen to the child with cerebral palsy. (*Hint:* Use the Drug Guide and see Chapter 49 in your textbook.)

9. List three side effects of this medication that place Stephanie at risk for personal injury.

• Click on **Consultations** and read the PT/OT Consult.

10. What specific therapy is recommended for Stephanie Brown by the physical therapist based on the findings during the consult?

11. What is an ankle-foot orthosis (AFO)? When did Stephanie Brown start wearing an AFO? State the purpose of the AFO. (*Hint:* See Therapeutic Management of Cerebral Palsy in Chapter 49 of your textbook.)

 • Click on **Nurse's Notes**.
 • Review the Nurse's Notes from the ED admission through Wednesday.

 12. What specific request does Stephanie Brown's mother make of the social worker? (*Hint:* Read the note on Tuesday at 1500.)

 13. Describe age-appropriate activities that can help Stephanie Brown cope with the anxiety associated with hospitalization and respiratory isolation.

 14. What recommendations could you give Stephanie Brown's mother to promote Stephanie's daily bowel movement? (*Hint:* See Constipation in Chapter 41 of your textbook.)

- Click on **Return to Nurses' Station**.
- Click on **304** at the bottom of the screen to go to Stephanie Brown's room.
- Click on **Patient Care** and then on **Nurse-Client Interactions**.
- Select and view the video titled **1530: Preventive Measures**. (*Note:* Check the virtual clock to see whether enough time has elapsed. You can use the fast-forward feature to advance the time by 2-minute intervals if the video is not yet available. Then click on **Patient Care** and **Nurse-Client Interactions** to refresh the screen.)

15. What specific recommendation does the physical therapist make to Stephanie Brown's mother on the consult note and during the video?